Responding in Mental Health–Substance Use

MENTAL HEALTH–SUBSTANCE USE

Responding in Mental Health–Substance Use

Edited by

DAVID B COOPER

Sigma Theta Tau International: The Honor Society of Nursing Award
Outstanding Contribution to Nursing Award
Editor-in-Chief, Mental Health and Substance Use
Author/Writer/Editor

Radcliffe Publishing
London • New York

Radcliffe Publishing Ltd
33–41 Dallington Street
London
EC1V 0BB
United Kingdom

www.radcliffepublishing.com

Electronic catalogue and worldwide online ordering facility.

British Library Cataloguing in Publication Data

A catalogue record for this book is available from the British Library.

ISBN-13: 978 184619 341 5

Typeset by Pindar NZ, Auckland, New Zealand
Printed and bound by Cadmus Communications, USA

Contents

Preface

Approximately six years ago Phil Cooper, then an MSc student, was searching for information on mental health–substance use. At that time, there was one journal and few published papers. This led to the launch of the journal *Mental Health and Substance Use: dual diagnosis*, published by Taylor and Francis International. To launch the journal, and debate the concerns and dilemmas of psychological, physical, social, legal and spiritual professionals, Phil organised a conference for Suffolk Mental Health NHS Trust and Taylor and Francis. The response was excellent. An occurring theme was that more information, knowledge and skills were needed – driven by education and training.

Discussion with international professionals indicated a need for this type of educational information and guidance, in this format, and a proposal was submitted for one book. The single book progressed to become a series of six! The concept is that each book will follow on from the other to build a sound basis – as far as is possible – about the important approaches to mental health–substance use. The aim is to provide a 'how to' series that will be interactive with case studies, reflective study and exercises – you, as individuals and professionals, will decide if this has been achieved.

So, why do we need to know about mental health–substance use? International concerns related to interventions, and the treatment of people experiencing mental health–substance use problems, are frequently reported. These include:

➢ 'the most challenging clinical problem that we face'[1]
➢ 'substance misuse is usual rather than exceptional amongst people with severe mental health problems'[2]
➢ 'Mental health and substance use problems affect every local community throughout America'[3]
➢ 'The existence of psychiatric comorbidities in young people who abuse alcohol is common, especially for conditions such as depression, anxiety, bipolar disorder, conduct disorder and attention-deficit/hyperactivity disorder'[4]
➢ 'Mental and neurological disorders such as depression, schizophrenia, epilepsy and substance abuse . . . cause immense suffering for those affected, amplify people's vulnerability and can lead individuals into a life of poverty'.[5]

There is a need to appreciate that mental health–substance use is now a concern for us all. This series of books will bring together what is known (to some), and what is not (to some). If undertaken correctly, and you, the reader will be the judge – and those individuals you come into contact with daily will be the final judges – each book will build on the other and be of interest for the new, and the not so new, professional.

The desire to provide services that facilitate best practice for mental health–substance use is not new. The political impetus for this approach to succeed now exists. We, the professionals, need to seize on this momentum. We need to bring about the much-needed change for the individual who experiences our interventions and treatment, be that political will because of a perceived financial benefit or, as we would hope, the need to provide therapeutic interventions for the individual. Whatever the motive, now is the time to grasp the initiative.

Before we (the professionals) can practise, research, educate, manage, develop or purchase services, we must commence with knowledge. From that, we begin to understand. We commence using our new-found skills. We progress to developing the ability to examine practice, to put concepts together, to make valid judgements. We achieve this level of expertise though education, training and experience. Sometimes, we can use our own life experiences to enhance our skills. But knowledge must come first, though is often relegated to last! Professionals (from health, social, spiritual and legal backgrounds) – be they students, practitioners, researchers, educators, managers, service developers or purchasers – are all 'professionals' (in the eye of the individual we meet professionally), though each has differing depths of knowledge, skills and expertise.

What we need to remember is that the individual (those we offer care to), family and carers bring their own knowledge, skills and life experiences – some developed from dealing with ill health. The individual experiences the illness, lives with it, manages it – daily. Therefore, to bring the two together, individual and professional, to make interventions and treatment outcome effective, to meet whatever the individual feels is acceptable to his or her needs, requires mutual understanding and respect. The professionals' skills and expertise '*are founded on nothing less than their complete and perfect acceptance of one, by another*'[6]

David B Cooper
January 2011

REFERENCES

1 Appleby L. *The National Service Framework for Mental Health: five years on*. London: Department of Health; 2004. Available at: www.dh.gov.uk/prod_consum_dh/groups/dh_digitalassets/@dh/@en/documents/digitalasset/dh_4099122.pdf (accessed 29 August 2010).

2 Department of Health. *Mental Health Policy Implementation Guide: dual diagnosis good practice guide*. London: Department of Health; 2002. Available at: www.substancemisuserct.co.uk/staff/documents/dh_4060435.pdf (accessed 29 August 2010).

3 Substance Abuse and Mental Health Service Administration. *Results from the 2008 National Survey on Drug Use and Health*. 2008. Available at: www.oas.samhsa.gov/nsduh/2k8nsduh/2k8Results.cfm (accessed 2 August 2010).

4 Australian Government. *Australian Guidelines to Reduce Health Risks from Drinking Alcohol.*

2009. Available at: www.nhmrc.gov.au/publications/synopses/ds10syn.htm (accessed 29 August 2010).

5 World Health Organization. *Mental Health Improvements for Nations Development: the WHO MIND Project.* World Health Organization; 2008. Available at: www.who.int/mental_health/policy/en (accessed 29 August 2010).

6 Thompson F. *Lark Rise to Candleford: a trilogy.* London: Penguin Modern Classics; 2009.

About the Mental Health–Substance Use series

The six books in this series are:
1 *Introduction to Mental Health–Substance Use*
2 *Developing Services in Mental Health–Substance Use*
3 *Responding in Mental Health–Substance Use*
4 *Intervention in Mental Health–Substance Use*
5 *Care in Mental Health–Substance Use*
6 *Practice in Mental Health–Substance Use*

The series is not merely for mental health professionals but also the substance use professionals. It is not a question of 'them' (the substance use professional) teaching 'them' (the mental health professional). It is about sharing knowledge, skills and expertise. We are equal. We learn from each fellow professional, for the benefit of those whose lives we touch. The rationale is that to maintain clinical excellence, we need to be aware of the developments and practices within mental health and substance use. Then, we make informed choices; we take best practice, and apply this to our professional role.[1]

Generically, the series Mental Health–Substance Use concentrates on concerns, dilemmas and concepts specifically interrelated, as a collation of problems that directly or indirectly influence the life and well-being of the individual, family and carers. Such concerns relate not only to the individual but also to the future direction of practice, education, research, service development, interventions and treatment. While presenting a balanced view of what is best practice today, the books aim to challenge concepts and stimulate debate, exploring all aspects of the development in treatment, intervention and care responses, and the adoption of research-led best practice. To achieve this, they draw from a variety of perspectives, facilitating consideration of how professionals meet the challenges now and in the future. To accomplish this we have assembled leading, international professionals to provide insight into current thinking and developments, from a variety of perspectives, related to the many varying and diverse needs of the individual, family and carers experiencing mental health–substance use.

REFERENCE

1 Cooper DB. Editorial: decisions. *Mental Health and Substance Use*. 2010; **3**: 1–3.

About the editor

David B Cooper
Sigma Theta Tau International: The Honor Society of Nursing Award
Outstanding Contribution to Nursing Award
Editor-in-Chief: *Mental Health and Substance Use*
Author/Writer/Editor

The editor welcomes approaches and feedback, positive and/or negative.

David has specialised in mental health and substance use for over 30 years. He has worked as a practitioner, manager, researcher, author, lecturer and consultant. He has served as editor, or editor-in-chief, of several journals, and is currently editor-in-chief of *Mental Health and Substance Use: dual diagnosis*. He has published widely and is 'credited with enhancing the understanding and development of community detoxification for people experiencing alcohol withdrawal' (Nursing Council on Alcohol; Sigma Theta Tau International citations). Seminal work includes *Alcohol Home Detoxification and Assessment* and *Alcohol Use*, both published by Radcliffe Publishing, Oxford.

List of contributors

CHAPTER 2   Professor Alex G Copello
Professor of Addiction Research and
Consultant Clinical Psychologist
School of Psychology/Addiction Services
University of Birmingham/Birmingham and Solihull Mental Health Foundation
Trust
Edgbaston
Birmingham, UK

Alex's career has combined clinical and academic work. His interests include the study of the impact of addiction upon families and the development and evaluation of family and social network-based interventions. Alex publishes regularly in scientific journals and has co-authored/edited: *Living with Drink: women who live with problem drinkers* (1998), *Substance Misuse in Psychosis: approaches to treatment and service delivery* (2002) (awarded a High Commendation in the 2003 BMA Book competition), *Cognitive Behavioural Integrated Treatment* (2004), *Coping with Alcohol and Drug Problems* (2005) and *Social Behaviour and Network Therapy for Alcohol Problems* (2009)

CHAPTER 3   Daren Garratt
Former Development Director
The Alliance
London, UK

Daren is the former Executive Director of the Alliance, a peer-led national charity that aims to improve the quality of drug treatment via the provision of a unique helpline service, specialist, independent advocacy, training and consultancy. Prior to working for the Alliance, Daren was DAT Coordinator for Walsall in the West Midlands, and a detached youth worker specialising in working with hard-to-reach users on the streets. Daren is a Director of the United Kingdom Harm Reduction Alliance (UKHRA), the drummer in the Nightingales, proud husband of Jez, and doting Dad to Ivy and Ruby.

Anthony A Birt
SevernSense Training and Consultancy Services
Formerly, Training Officer
The Alliance
London, UK

Tony was a regional advocate for the Alliance for three years before becoming its training lead for a year. He is currently working as a consultant and freelance trainer for SevernSense, a company he runs with his partner.

Linda Lee
Advocacy Manager
The Alliance
London, UK

Linda is the mother of two sons, one of whom has a severe dual diagnosis. She worked for Social Services for 23 years and has been working as an advocate for the Alliance for the last four years, so has experienced services as a provider and as a service user/carer.

CHAPTER 4   Jessica Davis
Chief Social Worker
Mid-West Area Mental Health Service
North Western Mental Health
Melbourne, Australia

Jessica is a Social Worker who has 10 years' experience mainly in the field of clinical mental health. However, Jessica has also worked within alcohol and other drug settings. Jessica has worked in academia lecturing and tutoring at both the University of Melbourne and La Trobe University. She has a strong commitment to the integrated care of those experiencing both a mental illness and substance use disorder and improving the health system to meet the needs of these consumers.

Professor Brenda M Happell
Professor of Contemporary Nursing
Department of Health Innovation and
Director, Institute for Health and Social Science Research
CQUniversity Australia
Rockhampton, Queensland
Australia

Brenda is an active researcher with a strong track record in publication, the supervision of higher degree students and obtaining competitive research funding. Her research interests include consumer participation in mental health services, seclusion, the physical health of people experiencing mental illness and mental health nursing education. Brenda is the editor of the *International Journal of Mental Health*

Nursing and a member of the board of directors of the Australian College of Mental Health Nurses.

Mikah Montgomery
Australia
Mikah is working as a consumer consultant in a public mental health service in Melbourne, Australia.

'It has been a long journey with my mental illness and drug and alcohol substance abuse situation. From 17 to 40, I was very sick, whereby I neglected my health, hygiene and fell into a lost abyss of daily scoring and living a broken record too. Since being diagnosed correctly with bipolar disorder and accepting my sentence, I have embraced professional help, medication and support from my carer, private psychiatrist and psychologist. I have developed as a person with natural leadership skills and acceptance by my peers and colleagues. I now look forward to a valued, productive, happy life.'

CHAPTER 5   Wayne Skinner
Deputy Clinical Director
Addiction programme
Center for Addiction and Mental Health
Assistant Professor, Department of Psychiatry
Adjunct Senior Lecturer, Faulty of Social Work
University of Toronto
Toronto, Ontario
Canada

Wayne edited *Treating Concurrent Disorders: a guide for counsellors* (2005) and co-authored (with Caroline O'Grady) *A Family Guide to Concurrent Disorders* (2007) and (with Marilyn Herie) *Substance Abuse in Canada* (2010). He is a member of the Motivational Interviewing Network of Trainers. He is Associate Editor (Canada) for the journal *Mental Health and Substance Use: dual diagnosis*.

Marilyn White-Campbell
Geriatric Addiction Specialist
Manager, Geriatric Mental Health Outreach Long Term Care
Community Outreach Program in Addiction (COPA)
Toronto, Ontario
Canada

Marilyn has worked with older adults with substance use and mental health issues with the COPA program – one of Canada's first addiction treatment programs for seniors – for over 24 years. She is considered a pioneer in the field of addictions/concurrent disorders and older adults. Marilyn is co-author (with Kate Graham *et al.*) of *Addictions Treatment for Older Adults: evaluation of an innovative client-centered approach.* Marilyn is on the International Advisory Board of Mental Health and Substance Use: dual diagnosis. She has presented nationally and internationally on the Canadian Model for Treatment of Older Adults with Substance Misuse.

Dr Helen MR Meier
Director, Psychogeriatric Services
Assistant Professor, Psychiatry
Dalla Lana School of Public Health
Mental Health and Addiction Program
St Joseph's Health Center
Toronto, Ontario
Canada

Helen began her medical education in Aberdeen, Scotland and continued in Psychiatry in London and Toronto, with an MSc in Psychiatric Epidemiology at University of Toronto and specialisation in Geriatric Psychiatry. An experienced educator, she works in community hospital settings with continuing focus on concurrent disorders (mental health and substance use), elder abuse and neglect and cultural dimensions of health/mental health, including services for immigrant and refugee care.

Dr Meldon Kahan
Associate Professor
Department of Family Medicine
University of Toronto
Medical Director
Addiction Medicine Service
St Joseph's Health Center
Toronto, Ontario
Canada

Meldon has written a number of peer-reviewed articles, guidelines and educational publications on addiction-related topics. His main interests are primary care and addiction, methadone and buprenorphine treatment, and medical education in addiction.

CHAPTER 6   Professor Ilana B Crome
Professor of Addiction Psychiatry and Academic Director of Psychiatry Consultant
Psychiatrist in Addiction
Academic Psychiatry Unit
Keele University Medical School
South Staffordshire and Shropshire Healthcare NHS Foundation Trust
Stafford, UK

Ilana is one of only three Professors of Addiction Psychiatry in the United Kingdom. Her interest and expertise in the field of comorbidity has informed the Department of Health and ACMD across the treatment, research and policy domains and this has been acknowledged by her appointment to the NICE Guideline Development Group on Mental Illness and Substance Misuse. She is a past President of the Alcohol and Drugs Section of the European Psychiatric Association, International Editor of the *American Journal on Addictions* and Joint Editor of *Drugs: Education, Prevention and Policy.*

Dr Alexander Baldacchino
Clinical Senior Lecturer in Addiction Psychiatry, University of Dundee
Consultant Psychiatrist in Addictions, National Health Service Fife
Director for the Centre for Addiction Research and Education Scotland (CARES)
Centre for Neuroscience, Division of Pathology and Neurosciences
Ninewells Hospital and Medical School
Dundee, Scotland

Alex has been researching comorbid substance misuse and associated psychiatric and physical issues for the last 15 years. His studies involved biological, neuropsychological, clinical and policy-related research. In the last 10 years, he has been the UK Principal Investigator to several European Union funded projects. These include looking at barriers and challenges faced by individuals with substance misuse-related problems accessing treatment (IATPAD Study), a cross-cultural multicentre study to determine the nature, extent and management of drug-related mental health problems in Europe (Drugs and Psychosis and ISADORA Studies) and the Internet and drug addiction (Psychonaut 2002 study) among others.

CHAPTER 7   Philip D James
Clinical Nurse Specialist in Child and Adolescent Substance Misuse
Youth Drug and Alcohol Services
Health Service Executive
Dublin, Ireland

Philip was appointed as the first Clinical Nurse Specialist in Child and Adolescent Substance Abuse in the Republic of Ireland in 2006 – a post he has maintained since. He trained as a psychiatric nurse in Dublin and in 2000 trained as a Rational Emotive Behavioural Therapist. Prior to taking up his current post he worked in a variety of adult mental health services. In addition to his clinical role, Philip has been involved in a variety of research projects and lectures on a variety of topics including substance abuse, borderline personality disorder and cognitive behavioural therapy.

Dr Bobby P Smyth
Consultant Child and Adolescent Psychiatrist
Youth Drug and Alcohol Service
Health Service Executive
Dublin, Ireland

Bobby has worked full-time with adolescents who have addiction problems for the past seven years in Dublin. He completed his higher specialist training in child psychiatry in Merseyside, England. He is a clinical lecturer with the Department of Public Health and Primary Care at Trinity College Dublin. He has been involved in addiction research for the past 15 years and has published over 20 addiction research papers in peer-reviewed journals on topics including addiction treatment outcome, unsafe injecting and alcohol abuse.

CHAPTER 8   Dr Victoria CL Manning
Honorary Lecturer
Institute of Psychiatry
National Addiction Centre
Psychological Medicine and Psychiatry
Institute of Psychiatry
London, UK
also
Research Manager, National Addictions Management Service
Institute of Mental Health
Adjunct Assistant Professor at Duke-NUS
Singapore

Victoria worked as a researcher for a decade, publishing over 30 peer-review papers in addiction. She is a chartered psychologist, holds a master's degree in health psychology and a PhD in neuropsychological functioning in patients with dual diagnosis. Other research interests include predictors of treatment outcome and peer-recovery networks. She is currently examining neuropsychological predictors of outcome for patients of addictive disorders in Singapore.

Dr Shai L van der Karre Betteridge
Consultant Clinical Neuropsychologist
City and Hackney NHS Community Health Service
Adult Community Rehabilitation Team
St Leonard's Hospital
London, UK

Shai is the clinical lead for Neuropsychology Rehabilitation Services, and has extensive experience and skills in neuropsychological assessment and cognitive rehabilitation with acquired brain injury and psychiatric populations. Shai has worked at a number of centres of excellence within the London region including the Wolfson Neurorehabilitation Centre, St George's Hospital, the Royal Hospital for Neuro-Disability, the Wellington Hospital and Broadmoor Hospital. She is also actively involved in clinical research exploring various aspects of cognitive rehabilitation, although primarily in relation to memory and executive dysfunction.

CHAPTER 9   Betty A Kitchener
Senior Lecturer
Orygen Youth Health Research Centre

Centre for Youth Mental Health
University of Melbourne
Parkville, Victoria
Australia

Betty is Program Director and co-developer of the Mental Health First Aid Training and Research Program. She has facilitated the spread of the Mental Health First Aid Program across Australia and to 15 other countries. Having experienced recurrent major depression herself, she brings an important consumer perspective to her work. Betty has received numerous awards for her Mental Health First Aid work, including an Exceptional Contribution to Mental Health Services Award and an Order of Australia Medal.

Professor Anthony F Jorm
Professorial Fellow
Orygen Youth Health Research Centre
Centre for Youth Mental Health
University of Melbourne
Parkville, Victoria
Australia

Anthony is a National Health and Medical Research Council Australia Fellow. His research focuses on public knowledge and beliefs about mental illnesses, and particularly on interventions to improve the public's helpfulness towards people developing mental illnesses. He is a co-developer of the Mental Health First Aid Program.

Dr Dan I Lubman
Professor of Addiction Studies and Services, Monash University
Director, Turning Point Alcohol and Drug Centre
Fitzroy, Victoria
Australia

Dan has worked across mental health and drug treatment settings in both the UK and Australia. Dan's research focuses on investigating substance use and comorbid mental health problems in youth. This includes the development of pharmacological and psychological treatment trials, as well as public health and school-based interventions.

CHAPTER 10   Dr Chris Holmwood
Director
Clinical Workforce Development and Standards
Drug and Alcohol Services South Australia
Clinical Services and Research
Parkside, Victoria
Australia

Chris has a background in general practice and for five years was the director of the South Australian Prison Health Service. He has particular clinical interests in the care of people with complex comorbidities, pain and substance dependence, as well as medical education and chronic disease management.

CHAPTER 11   Dr Hugh M Campbell

GP Principal and GP Specialist in Addiction Medicine
Harbour Drug and Alcohol Service
Plymouth Primary Care Addiction Service
Freedom Health Centre
Plymouth, UK

Hugh is a single-handed general medical practitioner in an inner-city area, and has 30 years' experience in a primary care setting. He is a general practitioner specialist in addiction medicine to the Plymouth primary care addiction service which receives referrals from local general practitioners. Hugh's MSc dissertation at St George's Hospital, London, kindled his interest in the presentation, assessment and treatment of patients with complex needs. Hugh collaborates closely with the local drug and alcohol service, addiction psychiatry and other mental health colleagues, and believes this special relationship is fundamental in providing a quality service to complex patients.

CHAPTER 12   Dr Brian R Rush

Senior Scientist and Co-Section Head
Health Systems Research and Consulting Unit
Centre for Addiction and Mental Health
Toronto, Canada

Brian holds a PhD in Epidemiology and Biostatistics and has worked for 33 years in a research and evaluation capacity in the substance abuse, problem gambling and mental health fields. Brian's research and development portfolio includes the field of co-occurring disorders with an emphasis on epidemiology in general and service populations, service- and system-level integration, and screening and assessment tools.

Dr Louise Nadeau
Professor
Département de Psychologie
Université de Montréal
Scientific Director
Centre Dollard-Cormier, University Institute on Dependencies
Associate Researcher
Douglas Mental Health University Institute, University McGill
Montréal
Québec, Canada

Louise's work focuses on alcohol and gambling, in particular on concurrent disorders and driving under the influence of alcohol. She is Chair of the boards of Éduc'alcool and the Canadian Foundation on Foetal Alcohol Research. She served as vice-chair of the Canadian Institutes of Health Research Governing Council (2000–2006). She was awarded the 2006 prix Marcel-Vincent for her work in the social sciences by ACFAS (the Francophone Association for Knowledge).

CHAPTER 13   Salena Williams

Senior Nurse Liaison Psychiatry
Department of Liaison Psychiatry
Bristol Royal Infirmary
Bristol, UK

Salena has worked as a psychiatric nurse for over 20 years. For the last eight years she has specialised in liaison psychiatry, working initially at the University Hospital of Wales, Cardiff, and currently at the Bristol Royal Infirmary. The psychiatric liaison team is multidisciplinary, and sees a range of psychiatric and comorbid conditions within the general hospital setting. As clinical team manager Salena oversees the work of the drug and alcohol specialist nurses within the hospital, as well as the psychiatric liaison team. Her specialist interest is the epidemiology and psychological aspects of suicide.

CHAPTER 14   Dr Lisa Blecha

Associate Practitioner
Addictology Centre
Centre de Recherché et de Traitment des Addictions (Centre of Addictions Treatment and Research)
Hopital Paul Brousse
Villejuif Cedex, France

Lisa is a practising addictologist and psychiatrist. She holds diplomas from Pierre and Marie Curie University and Descartes University, Paris. Her clinical duties include coordinating addictions care within a global treatment plan including hepatitis treatment and prevention. Her current research areas include psychiatric and somatic comorbidities in drug and alcohol-dependent patients, as well as genetic and environmental interactions in addictogenesis.

Dr Michael Lukasiewicz

Centre de Recherché et de Traitment des Addictions (Centre of Addictions Treatment and Research)
Hopital Paul Brousse
Villejuif Cedex, France

Michael is a practising psychiatrist and specialist in addictology. He holds a PhD from Pierre and Marie Curie University in Paris. He is a specialist in the area of psychiatric epidemiology in the prison environment and has numerous publications in the field.

Professor Michel Reynaud
Full Professor and Hospital Practitioner
Head, Department of Psychiatry and Addictology and Internal Medicine Pole
Centre de Recherché et de Traitment des Addictions (Centre of Addictions Treatment and Research)
Paul Brousse University Hospital
Villejuif Cedex, France

Michel is President of the French National College of Addictology Lecturers and coordinates several university diplomas and specialised training in addictology. Michel is also President of the French Addictology Federation and he was implicated in elaborating French psychiatric and addictology policy until 2000. Michel is the author and editor of over 20 textbooks for specialists including *A Treatise of Addictology* (Flammarion editions) and numerous national and international publications.

CHAPTER 15 Dr Cheryl Kipping
Consultant Nurse Dual Diagnosis
South London and Maudsley NHS Foundation Trust
University Hospital Lewisham
Lewisham, London, UK

Cheryl has provided dual diagnosis expertise to a variety of local and national advisory groups including the steering group that developed the Department of Health (2002) *Dual Diagnosis Good Practice Guide* and the NICE Guideline Development Group for Psychosis and Substance Misuse. Cheryl is one of the editors of the journal, *Advances in Dual Diagnosis*. To help achieve a work–life balance, she is a keen football supporter.

USEFUL CONTACTS Jo Cooper
Jo spent 16 years in Specialist Palliative Care, initially working in a hospice inpatient unit, then 12 years as a Macmillan Clinical Nurse Specialist. She gained a Diploma in Oncology at Addenbrooke's Hospital, Cambridge, and a BSc (Hons) in Palliative Nursing at The Royal Marsden, London, and a Specialist Practice Award. Jo edited *Stepping into Palliative Care* (2000) and the second edition, *Stepping into Palliative Care, Books 1 and 2* (2006), both published by Radcliffe Publishing. Jo has been involved in teaching for many years and her specialist subjects include management of complex pain and symptoms, terminal agitation, communication at the end of life, therapeutic relationships and breaking bad news.

Terminology

Whenever possible, the following terminology has been applied. However, in certain instances, when referencing a study and/or specific work(s), when an author has made a specific request, or for the purpose of additional clarity, it has been necessary to deviate from this applied 'norm'.

MENTAL HEALTH–SUBSTANCE USE

Considerable thought has gone in to the use of terminology within these texts. Each country appears to have its own terms for the person experiencing mental health and substance use problems – terms that includes words such as dual diagnosis, coexisting, co-occurring, and so on. We talk about the same thing but use differing professional jargon. The decision was set at the outset to use one term that encompasses mental health *and* substance use problems: *mental health–substance use*. One scholar suggested that such a term implies that both can exist separately, while they can also be linked.[1]

SUBSTANCE USE

Another challenge was how to term 'substance use'. There are a number of ways: abuse, misuse, dependence, addiction. The decision is that within these texts we use the term *substance use* to encompass all (unless specific need for clarity at a given point). It is imperative the professional recognises that while we may see another person's 'substance use' as misuse or abuse, the individual experiencing it may not deem it to be anything other than 'use'. Throughout, we need to be aware that we are working alongside unique individuals. Therefore, we should be able to meet the individual where he/she is.

ALCOHOL, PRESCRIBED DRUGS, ILLICIT DRUGS, TOBACCO OR SUBSTANCES

Throughout this book *substance* includes alcohol, prescribed drugs, illicit drugs and tobacco, unless specific need for clarity at a given point.

PROBLEM(S), CONCERNS AND DILEMMAS OR DISORDERS

The terms *problem(s)*, *concerns and dilemmas* and *disorders* can be used interchangeably, as stated by the author's preference. However, where possible, the term 'problem(s)' or 'concerns and dilemmas' had been adopted as the preferred choice.

INDIVIDUAL, PERSON, PEOPLE

There seems to be a need to label the individual – as a form of recognition! Sometimes the label becomes more than the person! 'Alan is schizophrenic' – thus it is Alan, rather than an illness that Alan lives with. We refer to patients, clients, service users, customers, consumers, and so on. Yet, we feel affronted when we are addressed as anything other than what we are – individuals! We need to be mindful that every person we see during our professional day is an individual – unique. Symptoms are in many ways similar (e.g. delusions, hallucinations), some need interventions and treatments are similar (e.g. specific drugs, psychotherapy techniques), but people are not. Alan may experience an illness labelled schizophrenia, and so may John, Beth and Mary, and you or I. However, each will have his/her own unique experiences – and life. None will be the same. To keep this constantly in the mind of the reader, throughout the book series we shall refer to the *individual*, *person* or *people* – just like us, but different to us by their uniqueness.

PROFESSIONAL

We are all professionals, whether students, nurses, doctors, social workers, researchers, clinicians, educationalists, managers, service developers, religious ministers – and so on. However, the level of expertise may vary from one professional to another. We are also individuals. There is a need to distinguish between the person with a mental health–substance use problem and the person interacting professionally (at whatever level) with that individual. To acknowledge and to differentiate between those who experience – in this context – and those who intervene, we have adopted the term *professional*. It is indicative that we have had, or are receiving, education and training related specifically to help us (the professionals) meet the needs of the individual. We may or may not have experienced mental health–substance use problems but we have some knowledge that may help the individual – an expertise to be shared. We have a specific knowledge that, hopefully, we wish to use to offer effective intervention and treatment to another human being. It is the need to make a clear differential, for the reader, that forces the use of 'professional' over 'individual' to describe our role – our input into another person's life.

REFERENCE

1 Barker P. Personal communication; 2009.

Cautionary note

Wisdom and compassion should become the dominating influence that guide our thoughts, our words, and our actions.[1]

Never presume that what you say is understood. It is essential to check understanding, and what is expected of the individual and/or family, with each person. Each person needs to know what he/she can expect from you, and other professionals involved in his/her care, at each meeting. Jargon is a professional language that excludes the individual and family. Never use it in conversation with the individual, unless requested to do so; it is easily misunderstood.

Remember, we all, as individuals, deal with life differently. It does not matter how many years we have spent studying human behaviour, listening and treating the individual and family. We may have spent many hours exploring with the individual his/her anxieties, fears, doubts, concerns and dilemmas, and the illness experience. Yet, we do not know what that person really feels, how he/she sees life and ill health. We may have lived similar lives, experienced the same illness but the individual will always be unique, each different from us, each independent of our thoughts, feelings, words, deeds and symptoms, each with an individual experience.

REFERENCE

1 Matthieu Ricard. As cited in: Föllmi D, Föllmi O. *Buddhist Offerings 365 Days*. London: Thames and Hudson; 2003.

Acknowledgements

I am grateful to all the contributors for having the faith in me to produce a valued text and I thank them for their support and encouragement. I hope that faith proves correct. Thank you to those who have commented along the way, and whose patience has been outstanding. Thank you to Jo Cooper, who has been actively involved with this project throughout – supporting, encouraging, listening and participating in many practical ways. Jo is my rock who looks after me during my physical health problems, and I am eternally grateful.

Many people have helped me along my career path and life – too many to name individually. Most do not even know what impact they have had on me. Some, however, require specific mention. These include Larry Purnell, a friend and confidant who has taught me never to presume – while we are all individuals with individual needs, we deserve equality in all that we meet in life. Thanks to Martin Plant (who sadly died in March 2010), and Moira Plant, who always encouraged and offered genuine support. Phil and Poppy Barker, who have taught me that it is OK to express how I feel about humanity – about people, and that there is another way through the entrenched systems in health and social care. Keith Yoxhall, without whose guidance back in the 1980s I would never have survived my 'Colchester work experience' and the dark times of institutionalisation, or had the privilege to work alongside the few professionals fighting against the 'big door'. He taught me that there was a need for education and training, and that this should be ongoing – also that the person in hospital or community experiencing our care sees us as 'professional' – we should make sure we act that way. Thank you to Phil Cooper, who brought the concept of this book series to me via a conference to launch the journal Mental Health and Substance Use: dual diagnosis, of which he was editor. It was then I realised that despite all the talk over too many years of my professional life, there was still much to be done for people experiencing mental health–substance use problems. Phil is a good debater, friend and reliable resource for me – thank you.

To Gillian Nineham of Radcliffe Publishing, my sincere thanks. Gillian had faith in this project from the outset and in my ability to deliver. Her patience is immeasurable and, for that, I am grateful. Thank you to Michael Hawkes and Jessica Morofke for putting up with my too numerous questions! Thank you to Jamie Etherington, Editorial Development Manager, and Dan Allen of the book marketing department, both competent people who make my work look good. Thanks also to Mia Yardley, Natalie Mason, Camille Lowe and the production team at Pindar,

New Zealand, for bringing this book to publication, and the many others who are nameless to me as I write but without whom these books would never come to print; each has his/her stamp on any successes of this book.

My sincere thanks to all of you named, and unnamed, my friends and colleagues along my sometimes broken career path: those who have touched my life in a positive way – and a few, a negative way (for we can learn from the negative to ensure we do better for others).

A final heartfelt statement: any errors, omissions, inaccuracies or deficiencies within these pages are my sole responsibility.

Dedication

This book is dedicated to Marc and Vicky. If one could parcel Marc's work, dedication, enthusiasm and compassion in animal welfare science and apply this to the field of mental health–substance use, the world would be a better place. Compassion is integral to Marc, which shows in everything he says and his actions. Humility is also a main strongpoint and something to be admired. Vicky's world is insurance, to which she is recently promoted, and dedicated. She is supportive of Marc's work dedication and ethic. Marc is also my son! Of whom, I am justifiably very proud.

CHAPTER 1

Setting the scene

David B Cooper

It seems that when problems arise our outlook becomes narrow.[1]

INTRODUCTION

The difficulties encountered by people who experience mental health–substance use problems are not new. The individual using substances presenting to the mental health professional can often encounter annoyance and suspicion. Likewise, the person experiencing mental health problems presenting to the substance use services can encounter hostility and hopelessness. 'We cannot do anything for the substance use problem until the mental health problem is dealt with!' The referral to the mental health team is returned: 'We cannot do anything for this person until the substance use problem is dealt with!' Thus, the individual is in the middle of two professional worlds and neither is willing to move, and yet, both professional worlds are involved in 'caring' for the individual.

For many years, it has been acknowledged that the two parts of the caring system need to work as one. However, this desire has not developed into practice. Over recent years, this impetus has changed. There is now a drive towards meeting the needs of the individual experiencing mental health–substance use problems, pooling expertise from both sides. Moreover, there is an international political will to bring about change, often driven forward by a small group of dedicated professionals at practice level.

Some healthcare environments have merely paid lip service, ensuring the correct terminology is included within the policy and procedure documentation, while at the same time doing nothing, or little, to bring about the changes needed at the practice level to meet the needs of the individual. Others have grasped the drive forward and have spearheaded developments at local and national level within their country to meet such needs. It appears that the latter are now succeeding. There is a concerted international effort to improve the services provided for the individual, and a determination to pool knowledge and expertise. In addition, there is the ability of these professional groups to link into government policy and bring about the political will to support such change. However, this cannot happen overnight. There are major attitudinal changes needed – not least at management and practice level.

One consultant commented that to work together with mental health–substance use problems would be too costly. Furthermore, the consultant believed it would create 'too much work'! Consequently, there is a long way to go – but a driving force to succeed exists.

Obtaining in-depth and knowledgeable text is difficult in new areas of change. One needs to be motivated to trawl a broad spectrum of work to develop a sound grounding – the background detail that is needed to build good professional practice. This is a big request of the hard-worked and pressured professional. There are a few excellent mental health–substance use books available. However, this series of six books is groundbreaking, in that each presents a much needed text that will introduce the first, but vital, step to the interventions and treatments available for the individual experiencing mental health–substance use concerns and dilemmas.

These books are educational. However, they will make no one an expert! In mental health–substance use, there is a need to initiate, and maintain, education and training. There are key principles and factors we need to bring out and explore. Some we will use – others we will adapt – while others we will reject. Each book is complete. Conversely, each aims to build on the preceding book. However, books do not hold all the answers. Nothing does. What is hoped is that the professional will participate in, and collaborate with, each book, progressing through each to the other. Along the way, hopefully, the professional will enhance existing knowledge or develop new concepts to benefit the individual.

The books offer a first step, relevant to the needs of professionals – at practice level or senior service development – in a clear, concise and understandable format. Each book has made full use of boxes, graphs, tables, figures, interactive exercises, self-assessment tools and case studies – where appropriate – to examine and demonstrate the effect mental health–substance use can have on the individual, family, carers and society as a whole.

A deliberate attempt has been made to avoid jargon, and where terminology is used, to offer a clear explanation and understanding. The terminology used in this book is fully explained at the beginning of the book, before the reader commences with the chapters. By placing it there the reader will be able to reference it quickly, if needed. Specific gender is used, as the author feels appropriate. However, unless stated, the use of the male/female gender is interchangeable.

BOOK 3: RESPONDING IN MENTAL HEALTH AND SUBSTANCE USE

As mentioned in the preface, the ability to learn and gain new knowledge is the way forward. As professionals we must start with knowledge, and from there we can begin to understand. We commence using our new-found skills, progressing to developing the ability to examine practice, to put concepts together and to make valid judgements.[2] This knowledge is gained through education, training and experience, sometimes enhanced by own life experiences.

Those we offer care to, and their family members, also bring their own knowledge, skills and life experiences, some developed from dealing with ill health. Therefore, making interventions and treatment outcome effective requires mutual understanding and respect.

In the book, primarily we:

➤ explore the comprehensive concerns and dilemmas occurring from, and in, mental health–substance use

➤ inform, develop and educate by sharing knowledge and enhancing expertise in this fast-developing interrelated experience of psychological, physical, social, legal and spiritual need.

We need to appreciate and understand the concerns and dilemmas that face the person before he/she comes to the service and professional for intervention and treatment. We have to adapt the service to respond to those individual needs. It is important to remember that each person is unique. Yes, there may be similarities in symptoms, and specific needs addressed for sex and age. However, we must accept and acknowledge that each will have variations and specific needs that have to be considered when developing appropriate services, and when interacting with the individual. Moreover, we must be aware of the needs of the family and carer who have their own specific needs.

This book gives grounding to the needs of the individual and family. Specifically, it will address the different needs by age and sex, and the types of responses that can be offered. Throughout, the book takes a person-centred approach and explores how we might adapt the responses to meet the individuals needs. It covers the ways in which different professionals come into contact with individuals and how to respond and manage various situations.

Chapters 2 to 7 look specifically at the following perspectives to be considered when developing care and interacting with the individual and family:

➤ family
➤ female
➤ older adult
➤ young person
➤ child.

For the female and family, stigma is important. Society is less tolerant of the female experiencing mental health–substance use problems. The older adult and young person have specific needs in relation to tolerance of substances. For the young person, recreational substance use and mental health can have major impact on the welfare of the individual. The older adult brings a unique set of concerns developed around bereavement, loss of status, loneliness and the lower level of substance tolerance. Moreover, the interaction between prescribed medication and mental health–substance use is a prominent concern. For the child there is a double concern in relation to the mental health–substance use of the parent or guardian and in terms of the child's own mental health and substance use.

We must also consider the effect of mental health–substance use on cognitive impairment for all age groups and adapt the service to meet the needs of the individual rather than expect the individual to meet the needs of the service. This is addressed in Chapter 8.

After exploring the needs of the individual by sex and age, Chapters 9 and 10 move on to explore the role of first aid and the general practitioner. These are the front line of intervention and treatment. Getting services and treatment right here can have a major impact on the future, and continuing well-being, of the individuals and family.

There is a continued debate around how much services should be integrated. In Chapter 12, Brian Rush and Louise Nadeau look at the issues surrounding service integration and planning. As an important debate, this offers an in-depth appreciation of the concerns and dilemmas, from all sides, offering a balanced view of the issues and opens the debate for further discussion. The crux is that, whatever evolves, the paramount need is to make sure it meets the needs of the individual. This comes first in any service development – if a successful outcome is to be achieved. It is important to remember that while one service may work well in a given area it may be disastrous in another. Thus, one service does not fit all. The service may need to be adapted or indeed be scrapped – to start afresh. Whatever the aim, unless we involve the individual and family in the development of such services – and LISTEN – we *will* get it wrong.

Chapters 13 and 14 open the text to further explore the needs of the individual and professional in the emergency setting and in prison. Again these are unique to the individuals, and service providers need to adapt appropriate intervention to meet those needs.

Whatever the stage of intervention we need to communicate harm reduction. We must acknowledge that it is not always possible to stop substance use. Thus, it is incumbent on all of us to give best possible guidance on the safe use of substances. We need to be tolerant of the individual who is not yet ready to move into effective action. Leaving the door open is essential. Harm reduction offers that link with services while offering a way in to services when the individual is ready.

CONCLUSION

We must remember that there is a constant theme throughout in relation to the need for properly funded education and training, not just for the professional but also for the individual. Just as important, there is constant reinforcement of why we need to know about mental health–substance use. This book is aimed at the professional, educator, service developer, manager and student, for we all need to be aware of the unique needs of the individual if our practice, interventions and treatment provision is to be effective.

It is hoped that this book is helpful and informative. One would hope that we feel sufficiently stimulated to proceed, having extended and developed this grounding in mental health–substance use. We can build upon our knowledge using the 'To learn more' sections as a guide to further study and knowledge. As one enters each new area of knowledge, so understanding improves of what is needed – and what is not. Our understanding grows of how we can apply this knowledge in practice and service development. With that comes the ability to use an open, non-judgemental and accepting approach to the problems identified by the individual presenting for intervention, treatment, advice or guidance.

Our knowledge and understanding constantly change. The challenge is to remain open and accessible to the knowledge and information that will help each of us provide appropriate therapeutic interventions:

➤ at the appropriate level of expertise

> at the appropriate time
> at the appropriate level of understanding of the individual, and her/his presenting concerns and dilemmas
> at the appropriate cost.

We cannot afford to be solid in the belief that all individuals are the same. If this book encourages us to be wise and flexible in practice and the development and provision of services, it has achieved its aim. If it helps us to appreciate some of the problems encountered by the individual, family and carers, it has achieved its aim. We can bring about much-needed changes for the individual experiencing mental health–substance use problems.

> *Wisdom and compassion should become the dominating influence that guide our thoughts, our words, and our actions.*[3]

REFERENCES

1 The 14th Dalai Lama. As cited in: Föllmi D, Föllmi O. *Buddhist Offerings 365 Days*. London: Thames and Hudson; 2003.

2 Bloom BS, Hastings T, Madaus G. *Handbook of Formative and Summative Evaluation*. New York, New York: McGraw-Hill Book Company; 1971.

3 Matthieu Ricard. As cited in: Föllmi D, Föllmi O. *Buddhist Offerings 365 Days*. London: Thames and Hudson; 2003.

The family perspective

Alex G Copello

Living with mental health–substance use problems in the family is highly stressful.

INTRODUCTION

Mental health and substance use problems, whether they occur separately or combined, have traditionally been studied by focusing mainly on the individual with the problems. Little attempt has been made to understand the social context within which these problems occur including the most immediate social environment that involves the family. On the whole, both research and treatment interventions have focused on variables or characteristics that are posited to be present within the individual and are seen as central to the development and course of the problems (e.g. biological make-up, psychological factors, etc.).

Those reading this chapter will be faced with two main challenges. The first is to think about mental health and substance use problems as an interactive pattern of experiences rather than two separate problems or 'conditions'. The second is to understand these experiences within a family context with less of an emphasis on individual variables of the person with the mental health–substance use problem, and more on the family experience and the family interactions.

When facing this challenge, however, we are to some extent limited by the available literature. Historically, there have been a number of both theoretical and practical attempts at understanding the experiences of families in both the substance use and the mental health fields. The latter two areas, however, have mostly developed in parallel with the exception of some more recent attempts at exploring the impacts of the combined mental health and substance use problems, or an earlier attempt to look at commonalities in family coping across a range of different conditions, including for example addiction, mental health, dementia and brain injury.[1] Overall, integration of work between the mental health and substance use fields has been limited and both areas have on the whole developed as two separate enterprises.

This chapter will begin by discussing briefly some of the ideas and research findings in the mental health and substance use areas separately before moving towards some of the more recent studies. We shall attempt to integrate what we know about the experience of families when both problems co-occur, before finally discussing some implications for how to provide a response to these highly prevalent problems.

FAMILIES AND SUBSTANCE USE

KEY POINT 2.2

Even though each family is unique, we can identify a number of common experiences that are present for family members when a person develops a mental health–substance use problem.

Early theories of families and substance use tended to focus on the role that families were perceived to play in causing these 'disorders'. Some of these early theories are discussed in more detail elsewhere.[2,3] The emphasis then was very much on the deficits of family members that were perceived as leading to the development of a substance use problem. In the case of alcohol, early theories stressed the pathology of female partners of men with drinking problems.[4,5] In relation to drug problems, the emphasis was on parental deficits that were hypothesised to lead to the development of drug use in their offspring.

KEY POINT 2.3

Families attempt to respond to this stressful experience, although at times the experience can feel overwhelming.

Later theories rejected the notion that families were part of the cause of the problem and focused instead on psychological concepts to understand the experience of substance use within a family unit. A stress and coping paradigm has been used by a number of authors to understand the factors that emerge when a substance use problem arises in the family setting.[3] In summary, stress-coping models suggest that when substance use problems emerge in the family, family members, other than the individual concerned, experience stress that can be severe and in most cases last for some time. In response to the stress, family members may use a range of behaviours or coping responses. Each coping response is usually experienced as a dilemma for family members and is associated with potential advantages and disadvantages. The central idea, however, is that people facing substance use problems in the family have the capacity to cope with these situations much as one would attempt to cope with any difficult, challenging and complex task in life. Common ways of coping in the face of substance use with possible advantages and disadvantages have been mapped out through research,[6] and are illustrated in Box 2.1.

BOX 2.1 Three ways of responding to substance use problems

1 **Engaged**
'Standing up to it': These responses involve active interactions between the family members and the individual aimed to change the substance use behaviour.

Examples: 'Keeping a close eye on him/her'; 'pleading with him/her'; 'arguing about substance use'.

Possible advantage: May help the family member feel that they are doing something positive.

Possible disadvantage: It may increase stress.

2 **Tolerant**
'Putting up with it': Responses that remove the negative consequences of the substance use behaviour from the individual.

Examples: 'Giving her/him money even when the family member thought it would be spent on substances'; 'clearing up a mess'.

Possible advantage: May avoid conflict.

Possible disadvantage: The family member may feel they are being taken advantage of.

3 **Withdrawal**
'Withdrawing and gaining independence': Responses that attempt to put distance between the family member and the individual.

Examples: 'Avoided him/her as much as possible'; 'taking up old interests'; 'spending more time away from home'.

Possible advantage: May prevent the family member from becoming too involved or feeling exhausted'.

Possible disadvantage: The family member may feel that they are not attempting to deal with the situation.

In essence, models based on a stress and coping paradigm emphasise the interactions between family members and the users of substances that are in turn influenced by the particular history and development of the problem. Each family is seen as unique and as an interacting group of individuals attempting to adapt and respond to the highly stressful circumstances that emerge from the development of a significant substance use problem in one of its members. Stress and coping models have also been used to develop intervention strategies.[7,8]

FAMILIES AND MENTAL HEALTH PROBLEMS

The development of the thinking and research in the area of families and mental health problems shows a similar trend to that present in the substance use literature. Early theories of schizophrenia, for example focused on the potential role that the family environment had in the aetiology of the disorder. One study described how a number of people in the field had identified the family as an important 'cause' of the illness.[9] They also note that although these ideas were influential, the lack of any evidence to support them meant that some of the later theories moved away from the notion of families as a cause of the mental health problem.

The focus moved to study factors that were seen to be contributing to the maintenance of the problem. In the late 1950s, investigators found that people with schizophrenia, who returned to live with the family after treatment, showed a higher relapse rate than those who did not.[10] This gave impetus to research into the area of 'expressed emotion'. The concept of 'high expressed emotion' was used to describe family environments with high frequencies of criticism, hostility or over-involvement from family members towards the person with schizophrenia. These family environments were associated with higher rates of relapse than those where the level of 'expressed emotion' was low.[11] This line of research was very important and influential, although it mostly focused on the outcomes for the person with the mental health problems. There was less of an attempt to investigate and further understand the experience of family members; for example, the emotions expressed were not linked to the family member's experience of the problem, or the studies did not capture the full complexity of the interaction between family member and the person with the mental health problem. Research on 'expressed emotion' led to a number of family intervention models developed on the basis that relapse to schizophrenia could be reduced by minimising the level of 'expressed emotion' in the family. Subsequent systematic reviews have shown these to be effective.[12]

'EXPRESSED EMOTION' AND MENTAL HEALTH–SUBSTANCE USE

One study discussed two important themes related to 'expressed emotion'.[13] These two themes are of particular importance when considering families facing mental health–substance use problems. The first issue that they discuss is the likelihood that higher levels of 'expressed emotion' may be found in family members who are facing more difficulty in coping rather than reflecting an enduring trait. Coping difficulty may emerge as a result of greater burden, increased behavioural problems or having fewer options available for responding. From this point of view, 'expressed emotion' can be seen as a form of coping similar to emotional coping behaviours identified in substance use and described earlier.

The second theme that they discuss is that of attribution. Attribution refers to the belief that family members hold about the cause of the symptoms of their relative with the problem. Family members that view symptoms as within the control of the individual tend to show more critical comments as opposed to those who perceive the symptoms as part of an illness and not within the individual's control.[14] The theme of attributions in relation to mental health–substance use was later explored in an empirical study.[15] The authors studied two samples of 42 families, one facing mental health problems and the other mental health–substance use.[15] Findings from this study suggested that those family members of the individual with mental health–substance use tended to see the symptoms and difficult behaviours of the individual as more within his/her control (i.e. made an internal attribution) when compared to families facing mental health problems without substance use. Although, overall, there were no differences between the two groups in terms of overall 'expressed emotion', more family members of the mental health–substance use group were rated as hostile and rejecting. Furthermore, when content analysis was used, the results showed that it was particularly negative symptoms that were the target of more criticism. A subsequent study replicated the findings when comparing a group of family members facing mental health (n = 32) and one facing mental health–substance use (n = 36).[16] These two studies stress two very important points. First, that the interpretation of symptoms and problems of the relative with mental health–substance use by family members will have a significant impact on how they respond and subsequent family interactions. Second, the results suggest the need to incorporate an exploration of attributions when working with family members of people experiencing mental health–substance use problems.

MENTAL HEALTH–SUBSTANCE USE: THE FAMILY EXPERIENCE

Overall, when reviewing the evidence in mental health–substance use, the importance of the family in terms of affecting the course and outcomes of the problems is recognised and supported. Through the integration of research findings, we can put forward a number of conclusions about the experience of family members facing significant mental health–substance use in a member of the family unit. These are discussed below.

Based on available evidence, we can conclude that family members who are affected by the mental health–substance use problem of a relative are best seen as victims of stress, attempting to respond to these circumstances as opposed to playing a causal role in the development of the problems. Family members are often unprepared to face these experiences and will attempt to respond to these events, often with little knowledge or past experience on which to base decisions. Even though in certain situations, family members' responses may compound the problem, overall families are not a central cause of the problem but should mostly be seen as part of the solution and a positive influence.

SELF-ASSESSMENT EXERCISE 2.1

Time: 10 minutes
What common stressors might influence the well-being of the family?

As a family member, the experience will involve a significant amount of stress that is likely to be severe and enduring. Research from families affected by alcohol and drug problems,[3] and mental health and substance use,[17] suggests that the experience is likely to include a range of stressors including uncertainty, isolation, worry about the relative and the impact on the family as a whole. Box 2.2 illustrates in more detail some of the common experiences described by family members facing these problems. The uncertainty felt by family members is further complicated by the difficulty in making sense of the manifest behaviour and the reasons for the problems present. Two further important stressors include the individual's behavioural problems and treatment motivation.[17] It is important that work with families focuses on the discussion of motivation for treatment and for substance use change in line with more recent developments.[18] This discussion can form part of a psychoeducational package to support families understand the complex processes of substance use and change.

KEY POINT 2.4

Working with families can lead to positive outcomes.

BOX 2.2 Common stressors described by family members

- Individual not pleasant or easy to live with
- Worry about the individual's health
- Financial irregularities
- Impact on other members of the family
- Social life affected for the family member or the whole family
- Incidents, crises
- Violence
- Not having enough help/support to provide care for the individual
- Isolation: physical and emotional.

SELF-ASSESSMENT EXERCISE 2.2

Time: 15 minutes
- Consider the experiences and challenges that family members may face.
- As you consider, make a note of the things that could be helped by adopting a positive approach.

The experience of stress over significant periods often leads to a range of physical and psychological symptoms of ill health for the family member. These symptoms may include:

➤ worry
➤ difficulty concentrating
➤ lack of sleep
➤ sickness
➤ loss of appetite
➤ low mood
➤ general anxiety symptoms.

It is not uncommon for family members to put up with these symptoms and receive little help and support. Coming forward and asking for help may feel like a significant step and take considerable time. In some cases, treatments will be offered for the symptoms (e.g. anxiety, depression) without an attempt to understand the underlying cause. Experiencing a range of complex emotions will also be part of the picture. These may include anger, shame and guilt.

Attempting to respond to the situation will involve difficult dilemmas for the family member, each potential response being associated with possible advantages and disadvantages. The alcohol and drug literature suggests that family member responses are usually influenced by thoughts and emotions.[19] Furthermore, in the case of people experiencing mental health problems, as well as substance use problems, the dilemmas are further complicated by the influence of attributions of symptoms by family members, and the impact that these attributions make on the interactions between family members and the person experiencing mental health–substance use problems.[15,16]

How family members respond will in turn affect the individual in a range of ways including potential engagement with treatment services and the level of substance use. A conceptual model, that incorporates family member stressors and well-being, and the impact that they have on the family members involvement with the person with mental health–substance use problems, as well as family member readiness to be involved in treatment, has been developed.[17] These factors in turn are hypothesised to influence the outcomes of the individual experiencing mental health–substance use problems, with positive engagement leading to improved outcomes.

One important aspect when reviewing the evidence is that people can change, and the patterns of interactions are not fixed. This is important when considering interventions to help people with mental health–substance use problems and their families. A family environment that may be critical and hostile at some stage could be changed into a more supportive environment, provided work is carried out to explore thoughts, emotions and attributions that are influencing particular types of interactions.

MENTAL HEALTH–SUBSTANCE USE IN THE FAMILY: PROVIDING A HELPFUL RESPONSE

It is important for professionals to respond in a positive way to families experiencing mental health–substance use problems. The first step in order to provide a response is to be familiar with the type of experiences and challenges that family members may face. An effective response will be important for two related reasons:
1 In order to reduce stress for the family member and the family as a whole.
2 To improve the likelihood of a good outcome for the person experiencing mental health–substance use problems.

Family approaches have been developed. Most commonly, the approaches described in the literature aim to engage the family member in the intervention for the person with the mental health–substance use problem. Some of the key components of the approaches described in the literature[20–22] are summarised in Box 2.3. It is important that the complexity of the situation is explored in a non-judgemental way and that strategies to respond are discussed in some depth, while support is offered to family members.

BOX 2.3 Important components of a positive response to families affected by mental health–substance use

- Practical advice and support (e.g. benefits)
- Education on mental health and substance use
- Impact of different substances
- Discuss and explore motivation and change process
- Explore family's coping responses and dilemmas
- Help families identify early signs and relapse cycles
- Encourage alternative activities
- Goal setting and problem-solving
- Explore support available for families.

SELF-ASSESSMENT EXERCISE 2.3

Time: 15 minutes

As the professional involved, what might you consider the important aspects to explore?

CONCLUSION

We can suggest that family members benefit from support in their own right. Brief structured interventions for family members have included:

➤ provision of information
➤ exploration of current coping
➤ development of support.

These have been effective in reducing stress for family members, and at the same time create less stressful family environments for all concerned.[7]

Family members need to maintain a delicate balance, experiencing some degree of control over the situation, while accepting that some of the behaviour may be an inevitable result of the mental health problem, and to maintain an atmosphere supportive of change.[16] This constitutes a dilemma. How to support families in this difficult task is the challenge for professionals.

REFERENCES

1 Orford J, editor. *Coping with Disorder in the Family*. London: Croom Helm; 1987.
2 Hurcom C, Copello A, Orford J. The family and alcohol: effects of excessive drinking and conceptualisation of spouses over recent decades. *Journal of Substance Use and Misuse*. 2000; **35**: 473–502.

3 Orford J, Natera G, Copello A, *et al*. *Coping with Alcohol and Drug Problems: the experiences of family members in three contrasting cultures*. London: Brunner-Routledge; 2005.

4 Whalen T. Wives of alcoholics: four types observed in a family service agency. *Quarterly Journal of Studies on Alcohol*. 1953; **39**: 632–41.

5 Futterman S. Personality trends in wives of alcoholics. *Journal of Psychiatric Social Work*. 1953; **23**: 37–41.

6 Orford J, Natera G, Davies J, *et al*. Tolerate, engage or withdraw: a study of the structure of families coping with alcohol and drug problems in South-West England and Mexico City. *Addiction*. 1998; **93**: 1799–813.

7 Copello A, Templeton L, Krishnan M, *et al*. A treatment package to improve primary care services for relatives of people with alcohol and drug problems. *Addiction Research*. 2000; **8**: 471–84.

8 Copello A, Templeton L, Velleman R, *et al*. The relative efficacy of two primary care brief interventions for family members affected by the addiction problem of a close relative: a randomised trial. *Addiction*. 2009; **104**: 49–58.

9 Barrowclough C, Tarrier N. *Families of Schizophrenic Patients: cognitive behavioural intervention*. London: Chapman and Hall; 1992.

10 Brown G, Carstairs G, Topping G. Post hospital adjustment of chronic mental health patients. *Lancet*. 1958; **2**: 685–9.

11 Bebbington P, Kuipers L. The predictive utility of expressed emotion in schizophrenia: an aggregate analysis. *Psychological Medicine*. 1994; **24**: 707–18.

12 Pitschel-Walz G, Leucht S, Bauml J, *et al*. The effect of family intervention on relapse and re-hosptalisation in schizophrenia: a meta-analysis. *Schizophrenia Bulletin*. 2001; **27**: 73–92.

13 Birchwood M, Jackson C. *Schizophrenia*. Sussex: Psychology Press; 2001.

14 Weisman A, Neuchterlein K, Goldstein M, *et al*. Expressed emotion, attributions and schizophrenia symptoms dimensions. *Journal of Abnormal Psychology*.1998; **2**: 355–9.

15 Barrowclough C, Ward J, Wearden A, *et al*. Expressed emotion and attributions in relatives of schizophrenia patients with and without substance misuse. *Social Psychiatry Epidemiology*. 2005; **40**: 884–91.

16 Niv N, Lopez SR, Glynn SM, *et al*. The role of substance use in families' attributions and affective reactions to their relative with severe mental illness. *Journal of Nervous and Mental Disease*. 2007; **195**: 307–14.

17 Townsend AL, Biegel DE, Ishler KJ, *et al*. Families of persons with substance use and mental disorders: a literature review and conceptual framework. *Family Relations*. 2006; **55**: 473–86.

18 Miller W, Rollnick S. *Motivational Interviewing: preparing people for change*. 2nd ed. New York: Guilford Press; 2002.

19 Orford J. Empowering family and friends: a new approach to the secondary prevention of addiction. *Drug and Alcohol Review*. 1994; **13**: 417–29.

20 Barrowclough C. Family intervention for substance misuse in psychosis. In: Graham HL, Copello A, Birchwood M, *et al*., editors. *Substance Misuse in Psychosis*. Chichester: Wiley; 2003. pp. 227–43.

21 Graham H, Copello A, Birchwood M, *et al*. *Cognitive-Behavioural Integrated Treatment*. Chichester: Wiley; 2004.

22 Smith G, Gregory K, Higgs A. *Integrated Approaches to Family Interventions: a manual for practice*. London: Jessica Kingsley Publishers; 2007.

TO LEARN MORE

- Smith G, Gregory K, Higgs A. *Integrated Approaches to Family Interventions: a manual for practice*. London: Jessica Kingsley Publishers; 2007.
- Graham H, Copello A, Birchwood M, *et al*. *Cognitive-Behavioural Integrated Treatment*. Chichester: Wiley; 2004.
- Barrowclough C. Family intervention for substance misuse in psychosis. In: Graham HL, Copello A, Birchwood M, *et al.*, editors. *Substance Misuse in Psychosis*. Chichester: Wiley; 2003. pp. 227–43.
- **Useful website for family members**: www.dualdiagnosis.co.uk/TalkingHeads.ink ('What it means to make a difference: caring for people with mental illness who use alcohol and drugs')

CHAPTER 3

The individual's perspective: hard to reach people or hard to access services?

Daren Garratt, Anthony A Birt and Linda Lee

PRE-READING EXERCISE 3.1

Time: 15 minutes
- Individuals experiencing mental health–substance use problems are 'hard to reach', almost certainly 'hard to hear', clearly 'hard to attract', and invariably 'hard to please'. But are they really that 'hard to cater for'?
- What are the factors that make these individuals so problematic to service providers?
- Consider your answer from the individual's and agency perspectives.

What do we mean by this term 'hard to reach'? Is it fair or appropriate that in this first decade of the 21st century we continue to peddle the implication that because the majority of people accessing services are white, male (presumably heterosexual), using opiates, in the 18–35 age range, anyone who falls outside of this profile is somehow difficult? That they are 'hard to reach' because specific considerations that are shaped or influenced by their individual needs, politics, gender, culture, age and heritage are not reflected in the systems we have inherited, promote and still work within.

Is this not – in essence – just a further extension of the blame culture that still underpins whole swathes of drug treatment provision in the UK; the 'problematic' substance use, the 'chaotic' lifestyle, the 'difficult' individual, the 'hard to reach' group? Perhaps only when we begin to talk of the 'problematic' treatment regime, the 'chaotic' bureaucracy, the 'difficult' provider and the 'hard to access' service in equal measures will we be at a point where we can work effectively and constructively to redress this balance.

However, where do people experiencing mental health–substance use problems fit in to this category? Why are they viewed as particularly 'hard to reach'?

'Substance misuse is usual rather than exceptional amongst people with severe mental health problems and the relationship between the two is complex. Individuals with these dual problems deserve high quality, patient-focused, integrated care. These should be delivered within mental health services.'[1]

One clear directive – *see* Key point 3.1 – states all we need to know on the subject, and puts the whole notion of individuals experiencing mental health–substance use issues as being somehow 'hard to reach' into question.

So, to summarise again:

➤ Substance use is common among people with mental health issues.

➤ High-quality, individualised, integrated care should be delivered.

➤ This is the responsibility of mental health services.

Yet still, the field is rife with examples of contradictory and potentially life-threatening malpractice that allows vulnerable individuals to fall between the cracks of service provision and to be denied the coordinated care to which they are entitled.

To quote Linda Lee, the Alliance's Advocacy Manager and long-time campaigner for mental health, drug use and criminal justice reform:

> If there is so much evidence that has been written, accepted and acknowledged by the Department of Health and other statutory organisations and recommendations for practice been made, why has this not been put into practice?
>
> The consequences are that the most severely ill and disadvantaged in our society are being failed by services. They either end up committing suicide or spending their lives in prison where they are segregated and locked up 24 hours a day as the prison staff and prison setting are not equipped to cope.[2]

So why are we still failing these individuals? What can we do to redress this imbalance?

ADVOCACY: THE ROLE AND IMPORTANCE IN RESOLVING ISSUES

'Advocacy is taking action to help people say what they want, secure their rights, represent their interests and obtain services they need. Advocates and advocacy schemes work in partnership with the people they support and take their side. Advocacy promotes social inclusion, equality and social justice.'[3]

Advocacy fits within drug treatment systems as an independent way of resolving problems where it has not been possible to resolve the problem informally between the individual and professional or agency. Independent advocacy services are those where the named advocate provides objective, evidence-based support and guidance to an individual who is at risk of experiencing isolation or conflict around an issue that could affect their life and well-being.

This is extremely pertinent when considering the problems and issues that many people experiencing mental health–substance use issues face, but how effective can an advocate be when the whole system appears to work against the individual's best interest?

Case study 3.1 Part I

Jenny and her partner George live within the borders of two counties. Jenny has been using amphetamines for years, as has her partner. It is their 'drug of choice'. George is concerned about Jenny and says that she uses base amphetamine and 'street' Dexedrine as often as possible, usually four or five times a week.

In the past, Jenny also used heroin, but she is now stabilised on substitute prescribing treatment.

Until recently, Jenny was being treated by her county Community Drug Team (CDT), but she left following an incident where she felt 'misrepresented' by her key worker at a meeting during which Jenny had asked her consultant to prescribe her Dexedrine.

Jenny states that her amphetamine use 'has never been addressed by the CDT'. During recent discussions with her key worker, Jenny was reassured that she should meet the criteria for Dexedrine prescribing. However, during the meeting with the consultant, Jenny was told that she would not be prescribed Dexedrine, as she did not fit the criteria. Jenny is still not aware what the criteria are.

Jenny is now being treated by the bordering county's CDT. She is receiving methadone and has a key worker. Jenny has approached the service about prescribing Dexedrine but they refused, as they felt that she was not an appropriate candidate.

Jenny is struggling to cope with her current lifestyle but continues to use amphetamines regularly. She feels very strongly that a prescription would help her to stabilise and work towards moving away from her dependence. Jenny would like to start a new life; she has ended past friendships and would like to meet new people.

Jenny's partner, George, was in a similar situation. He is currently being prescribed Dexedrine by Jenny's original CDT and has stopped all his illicit use. They are living together and this is putting further pressure on their relationship and their attempts to address their drug use.

Jenny suffered from a 'mental breakdown' four years ago and is concerned about her mental health and she is feeling very stressed by this situation. She feels confused by the whole situation and does not understand why she is not going to be considered for Dexedrine prescribing. The key worker and consultant have explained very little about the decision and Jenny would like to know more about it.

SELF-ASSESSMENT EXERCISE 3.1 – *SEE* P. 23 FOR ANSWERS

Time: 15 minutes
- What issues stand out?
- What are the 'complexities of the case'?
- What issues might people with different perspectives have?
- What is 'the debate'?

Case study 3.1 Part II

After a few weeks, Jenny called the advocate. She is feeling much worse and says that she just cannot carry on with the situation.

About a week ago, George started to share his Dexedrine prescription with Jenny when she was unable to get anything else. At first this was manageable but it soon became a more regular and then daily occurrence. Consequently, George is now also using illicit drugs. Jenny and George are both really struggling; the situation is affecting all aspects of their lives.

Recently the advocate has struggled to maintain contact with Jenny and this conversation helped to clarify why. Jenny seemed more emotional and less rational about the situation. Jenny apologised for not being around much recently and said, 'You know how it is; I'm just not very together at the moment.'

SELF-ASSESSMENT EXERCISE 3.2 – *SEE* PP. 23–24 FOR ANSWERS

Time: 15 minutes
- What effect could this situation have on Jenny and George?
- Does the new information change the advocate's understanding and/or approach?
- If so, how?

Case study 3.1 Part III

Following some months of waiting and preparation the advocate attended an appointment with Jenny, her key worker and the consultant. The appointment lasted for two and a half hours, during which time the consultant used the opportunity to listen to Jenny and to the reasoning of the advocate. However, the consultant was firm in his refusal to prescribe Dexedrine, but after further discussion around the personal and wider benefits of prescribing for Jenny the consultant conducted a basic psychiatric evaluation and agreed to the advocate's suggestion of prescribing under a contract.

SELF-ASSESSMENT EXERCISE 3.3 – *SEE* P. 24 FOR ANSWERS

> **Time: 15 minutes**
> What might the advocate suggest should/could be included in the contract?

Case study 3.1 Part IV

The consultant wrote the contract there and then and was reassured that Jenny felt happy to comply with all points specifically around reducing and stopping illicit amphetamine and Dexedrine use. Prescribing commenced on 30 mg of Dexedrine tablets a day, to be titrated up to around 50 mg if Jenny needed it, daily supervised consumption to begin with. Jenny was happy to sign the contract and the appointment ended on a high note.

The moral of the story is that, despite all factors pointing to the opposite – woman, stimulant user with history of mental health issues requires stimulant prescription – cases such as this can be resolved if approached in a methodical, evidence-based, common-sense way.

Jenny was not the problem; service policy was. However, with clear methodical planning, and understanding of various guidelines and best practice documents, the advocate was able to construct a clear, concise case that brought a successful resolution.

However, what happens when the individual presents with, arguably, more complex and pressing concerns than those of Jenny? The current, ongoing and seemingly intractable gulf between mental health and substance use treatment services still allows the most vulnerable individuals to be shunted between services, and fail to receive the integrated package of care they deserve and are entitled to.

These are real lives, a point we need to always bear in mind as we consider the ongoing, unresolved case of William.

Case study 3.2

William is a 32-year-old man experiencing mental health–substance use problems. He has a 10-year history of poly-drug use, including alcohol, and is opiate dependent. He has a history of chronic anxiety, homelessness and post-traumatic stress disorder, after incarceration for petty crime to fund his drug habit.

He has no history of violence. He has engaged with drug treatment several times and tried to engage with mental health services in the past, but they would not treat him because he used heroin.

William had an acute mental illness episode two years ago following an extremely traumatic event. He was floridly psychotic. This led to two suicide attempts and hazardous substance use. Mental health services finally engaged with him and he was sectioned under the UK Mental Health Act for an assessment period (28 days).

The psychiatrist had no basic drug education and told William that he used his mental health issues as an excuse to use drugs, that all drug users were the same, and that his illness was self-inflicted. William's mother and main carer had considerable knowledge and experience of drug treatment and understanding of her son's problems, but she was ignored by the psychiatric consultant.

The consultant decided to discharge William after 10 days against his mother's wishes and evidence as to the high risk her son presented. Two days later, he made his third suicide attempt, throwing himself off a cliff, falling 50 feet onto concrete. He fractured his skull, hip and facial bones, and damaged his spleen. He miraculously survived.

He had to wait in Accident and Emergency for 10 hours to be assessed by a psychiatrist. He was sectioned under the UK Mental Health Act two days after a hip operation and taken to a mental health ward. He could not move without assistance, could not walk and was placed in a room on the first floor with no wheelchair, a low, hard plastic mattress and with no equipment to aid mobility, no pain control or case notes.

William partially recovered physically, was discharged but relapsed to heroin use. He often refused to engage with mental health services in the community but began taking methadone again. There were further sections, and an involuntary discharge. This placed William in a high suicide risk category. He almost overdosed on heroin the first day and refused to engage with mental health services or take his medication.

William has been an informal patient on a mental health ward for nearly six months, but his symptoms are becoming worse. His delusions are treatment resistant. There is a local pub nearby and because William is not sectioned under the UK Mental Health Act he is free to visit the pub when he likes, which is usually about four times a week. He drinks about four to six pints of beer each time.

William has put on nearly 10 stone in a year. He has had no physical exploratory tests for head injury trauma. Nor has he been referred to a neuropsychiatrist or mental health–substance use professional.

He has inadequate pain relief for his hip and past toothache because his requests for pain control are seen as 'drug-seeking behaviour'.

His consultant and ward-based professionals have no training in drug treatment. When he asks for symptomatic relief for his anxiety it is refused, as again this is seen as 'drug-seeking behaviour'.

His consultant has tried to reduce William's methadone against his will because he does not understand the benefits.

There is no integrated working or mainstreaming services for mental health–substance use, nor are there any resources in the county.

An out-of-county placement at a specialist mental health–substance use resource has been refused at appeal.

REFLECTIVE PRACTICE EXERCISE 3.1

Time: 40 minutes
- What are the issues here?
- What are the implications for future treatment planning?
- What is your understanding of the term 'mental health–substance use'?
- How do you know who to approach when advocating for mental health–substance use practice when professionals do not know their own roles, responsibilities, policies, resources or governance?
- Where do you think training in mental health–substance use should be targeted?
- Why are 74% of people experiencing mental health–substance use problems in prison at a cost on average of £3500 a month? This is a setting where suicide is at least four times higher than in the community and these people require treatment not prison. These individuals are already high suicide risk.
- Why are these individuals being punished in inhumane conditions instead of treated?
- Why is this money not being transferred to community and health services so people can access the help they need in the community?

SELF-ASSESSMENT EXERCISE 3.4

Time: 10 minutes
- Where are the mental health–substance use services in your area?
- Where are the funding streams?

Purposefully, there are no answers given to Case study 3.2. Sometimes, the answer is in the not knowing but the exploring. These are the realities that *you*, the professional, have to consider. These realities face many individuals, their families and carers. They certainly do not have the answers!

CONCLUSION

As long as people with both mental health and substance use problems receive treatment of such variable quality, much work remains to be done. Mental health professionals need a deeper knowledge of substance use, substance use professionals need a deeper knowledge of mental health issues, and the advocate's role in raising the professionals' awareness and advocating on behalf of individuals will continue to be crucial.

However, many individuals, their families and carers have no easy answers to their problems. Even with the full support of an advocate, even with the support of well-informed drug and mental health professionals, some cases will always be intractable.

ANSWERS TO SELF-ASSESSMENT EXERCISES 3.1 TO 3.3

Q: What issues stand out?
- Mental health
- George and Jenny's relationship
- Cross-county working
- New Community Drug Team. Jenny does not know them; they do not know her
- Illicit drug use
- Stabilised on methadone script (maintaining the status quo)
- George being prescribed when Jenny is not – will probably cause issues for one or both.

Q: What are the 'complexities of the case'?
- Cross-county work
- Dexedrine prescribing not common
- Lack of guidance on the subject
- Varied approaches
- Prescribing and mental/physical health issues.

Q: What issues might people with different perspectives have? What is 'the debate'?
- It is not safe to prescribe Dexedrine to a person with mental health issues.
- Drug-use history (could be using heroin or going to – poly-drug use).
- Prescribing for dependence not physical addiction (Jenny does not *need* it).

Q: What effect could this situation have on Jenny and George?
- Relationship
- Financial
- Work
- Social
- Mental health
- Increased drug use (illicit and prescribed)
- Dilution of treatment (Jenny and George now getting inappropriate care/ treatment)
- Discharge from treatment for George.

Q: Does this new information change the advocate's understanding and/or approach? If so, how?
- Possible mental health episode (obvious confusion)
- Depression
- Emotional
- Anxiety
- Increased drug use
- George returning to drug use, George less stable
- More chaotic lifestyle, 'less together'
- Relationship difficulties (possible breakdown and less support)

- Not in regular contact with advocate (situation could be changing/is getting worse)
- Possibility of advocate concern that Jenny is no longer suitable for prescribing
- Advocate feels that a personal visit is necessary to get a better picture.

Q: What might the advocate suggest should/could be included in the contract?

- Agreed dose amount
- Daily and/or supervised consumption
- Not using street drugs
- Reduction regime
- Regular check-up and review
- Attendance at key work sessions
- Other engagement in services, e.g. specific counselling
- Signed and dated by both/all present.

REFERENCES

1 Department of Health. *Mental Health Policy Implementation Guide: dual diagnosis best practice guide*. London: Department of Health; 2002. p. 4.

2 Lee L. Personal communication; June 2010.

3 Action for Advocacy. *The Advocacy Charter*; 2004. Available at: www.aqvx59.dsl.pipex.com/Advocacy%20Charter2004.pdf (accessed 16 June 2010).

TO LEARN MORE

- Rethink and Turning Point's *Dual Diagnosis Toolkit*. www.rethink.org/dualdiagnosis/toolkit.html
- The Department of Health's *Dual Diagnosis Good Practice Guide*. www.dh.gov.uk/prod_consum_dh/groups/dh_digitalassets/@dh/@en/documents/digitalasset/dh_4060435.pdf
- The patient.co.uk definition of dual diagnosis: www.patient.co.uk/doctor/Dual-Diagnosis-(Drug-abuse-with-other-psychiatric-conditions).htm

CHAPTER 4

The female perspective

Jessica Davis, Brenda M Happell and Mikah Montgomery

INTRODUCTION

Co-occurring mental illness and substance use is the '*expectation not the exception*'[1] within either mental health or substance use treatment settings. Within clinical practice, professionals soon become aware of the grave challenge of treating mental illness–substance use problems and the chasm between the two service sectors and the disempowerment experienced by the individual, family and carers, often caught in between the two sectors.

Many who have worked within both settings, or either one, are frequently perplexed by the actions of some professionals who do not accept that in order to assist individuals experiencing a mental health–substance use disorder, integrated treatment is essential. Unless both issues are addressed concurrently, ideally by the same treating team, best outcomes will not be achieved.[2] Working within a system that has traditionally had mental health and substance use services operating in silos has often placed individuals with the burden of negotiating their treatment between two very different sectors. All too frequently, one sector passes the responsibility to the other.

Some positive developments are evident. For example, the Victorian Government in Australia has recognised the burden individuals, family and carer(s) face in regards to mental health–substance use and are trying to address these challenges through system, policy and workforce changes, in order to shift the burden to integrate care back to the system.

SERVICE DEVELOPMENT

The new initiative in service provision in Victoria, Australia, was signalled by the release of the *Dual Diagnosis: key directions and priorities for service development.*[3] The contents of this document provided an impetus for clinical mental health services, psychiatric disability support services and substance use services to treat the provision of service to the individual experiencing metal health–substance use disorders as '*core business*'. A set of Service Development Outcomes was set out with timelines attached to be completed by the end of 2010. These were as follows:

1 Dual diagnosis is systematically identified and responded to in a timely

evidence-based manner as core business in both mental health and alcohol and other drug services.

2   Staff in mental health and alcohol and other drug services are 'dual diagnosis capable', that is, have the knowledge and skills necessary to identify and respond appropriately to dual diagnosis clients, and advanced practitioners are able to provide integrated assessment, treatment and recovery.

3   Specialist mental health and alcohol and other drug services establish effective partnerships and agreed mechanisms that support integrated assessment, treatment and recovery.

4   Outcomes and responsiveness for dual diagnosis clients are regularly reviewed.

5   Consumers and carers are involved in the planning and evaluation of service responses.[3]

ISSUES OF GENDER

This policy document has opened a dialogue between mental health and substance use services that is a positive shift in the treatment paradigm, which will only prove positive for the individual experiencing mental health–substance use disorder. However, nowhere in the document does it mention the provision of services to women specifically, or address any issues of gender within the policy initiative. Why is this? Gender issues within mental health seem to be one of the last taboo areas. Is this a fiscal issue? Is this due to a lack of meaningful consultation? Or is it the spectre of the old institutions where care for those experiencing mental health issues was provided in separate wards? There is an argument for all of the above.

Deinstitutionalisation commenced in Australia in earnest in the late 1980s, where the closure of large psychiatric hospitals saw the shift of care for those with mental health and substance use issues to community care teams. Victoria, Australia, also witnessed the transfer of the guidance of substance use services to non-government organisations while clinical mental health services stayed within the domain of government-run services, establishing community clinics which were organisationally connected to psychiatric inpatient units attached to public hospitals. Prior to this there were many facilities that had psychiatric inpatient facilities and alcohol and other drug detoxification units on the same campus, sometimes down the hospital corridor from each other! Many of these units were also segregated by gender.

Later in this chapter Mikah will speak of the trauma she and other women have experienced when experiencing a relapse in either their mental illness or substance use, and the vulnerability experienced in a mixed gender unit when they are unwell. One study discusses the potential impact upon women who are admitted to psychiatric inpatient units, summarising a range of challenges which are specific to women, such as contraception, pregnancy care and sexual health.[4] These challenges can also be highlighted within alcohol and other drug detoxification units. The authors expand on these challenges by highlighting that the provision of acute inpatient care '*by definition can be disempowering for many women, in particular, the ways in which services are provided to trauma survivors may unintentionally trigger feelings of powerlessness and cause the individual to feel re-traumatized*'.[4] Exposure to traumatic behaviour, such as aggression, self-harm, use of illicit substances and seclusion or physical restraint of individuals can impact on those who have experienced trauma. '*Over one-third of service users have experienced physical assaults and up to two-thirds have witnessed traumatic events in psychiatric settings.*'[4] Of particular concern is the risk of sexual assault for women being cared for in an acute setting whether this is within the mental health or substance use sectors.

Mikah (*see* p. 30) speaks of feeling as if her expression of distress, which translated into psychotic relapses, heavy substance use and destructive behaviours, was treated by professionals as 'consequences she needed to take responsibility for' as opposed to evidence of her psychological distress.

> [C]linicians experience and judge such female behaviour as annoying, inconvenient, stubborn, childish, and tyrannical. Beyond a certain point, such behaviour is 'managed', rather than rewarded: it is treated with disbelief and pity, emotional distance, physical brutality, economic and sexual deprivation, drugs, shock therapy, and long-term psychiatric confinements.[5]

To translate this commentary into the current day, prison incarceration, homelessness and exploitative relationships are often the dysfunctional respite for women experiencing mental health–substance use problems.

This response from professionals combined with the health system's lack of sensitivity to the vulnerability of women who are undergoing detoxification and/or experiencing a mental illness as a whole can be interpreted within a feminist framework, such as Phyllis Chessler's controversial text *Women and Madness.*[6] Chessler discusses the expectations that psychiatry and the broader society have of women and their behaviour and consequent treatment within psychiatric facilities: '*Given the custodial nature of asylums and the anti-female biases of most clinicians, women who seek "help" or women who have "symptoms" are actually being punished for their conditioned and socially approved self-destructive behaviour.*'[5]

MOVING TOWARDS INDIVIDUALISED ENVIRONMENTS

Moves towards gender sensitive practice within mental health and substance use services are hindered by similar issues the individual faces in regards to tokenism and a lack of meaningful participation within service development; in this instance, women specifically. One article asserts that the role of the individuals within the development of service provision is pivotal to the future of mental health and substance use provision.[6] For groups with specific needs, such as women experiencing mental health–substance use disorders, this is particularly crucial. However, the article also warns about tokenism and calls for authentic involvement via the provision of clear articulated guidelines within the bureaucracy and key decision points within the infrastructure chain.[7] Although the development of 'women-friendly environments' or 'women-only sitting rooms' within psychiatric or substance use service settings are an acknowledgement of need, they are a small step to meaningful interpretation of women's treatment experiences being translated into the therapeutic milieu.

Outline barriers in relation to women seeking and remaining in treatment for substance use state that: '*these* [should] *include childcare issues, stigma and lack of support from others*'.[7] Co-occurring mental health and substance use is also cited as a contributing factor in women not completing alcohol and other drug treatment.[8]

Case study 4.1

James is a 33-year-old man with a diagnosis of schizophrenia and alcohol dependency. He has three children aged 2, 7 and 11 to three different women. None of the pregnancies was planned, but in each case James was excited by the news and made several attempts to stop drinking, with varying degrees of success. Between six months and two years after the birth of each child, James became progressively withdrawn, finding himself unable to cope with the responsibilities of parenting, fearing that he would hurt the baby and that the baby did not love him. The greater his fears and anxieties, the more he drank. His relationship with each of his partners deteriorated. James found the situation increasingly unbearable and eventually left. For a short while after leaving he attempted to keep in contact. Eventually, he either stopped because he found it too painful, or because his former partner told him to get out of their lives. James grieved the loss of his children. He was sad that he knew so little about them and would not be an important part of their lives, and felt they were better off without him. James finds it much easier to deal with his loss when he is drunk and has little motivation to give up drinking. He often has thoughts about ending his life 'for everyone's sake'.

SELF-ASSESSMENT EXERCISE 4.1

Time: 15 minutes
- How would you feel about the situation if James was female?
- Consider the role women have in society around childbearing and mothering
- Would your feelings around a female differ in the way they do to James?
- If so, how?

It is likely that many will consider James to be irresponsible and will consider his drinking and possibly his mental illness as a sign of weakness or avoidance. Change James to Janice and the response is likely to be much stronger. 'How could a woman do that to her children?' She would be described as uncaring, promiscuous, irresponsible and, worst of all, as unfit to be a mother. Women diagnosed with both a mental illness and substance use disorders are among the most marginalised and stigmatised people in our society.[9] These women will experience the discrimination associated with mental illness and with substance use. Being a woman makes what is difficult to understand in men virtually intolerable. Gender stereotypes allow men to engage in risqué behaviour but expect women to be 'lady-like, gentle and caring'.

Pregnancy and childbirth adds fuel to the fire. The woman who abandons the ultimate feminine responsibility of childbearing and rearing is considered beyond contempt. In some quarters the presence of mental illness might arouse some sympathy or understanding, but this is much less likely with substance use, which is generally interpreted as a sign of weakness or lack of responsibility. Often women take on these stigmatising attitudes, by feeling guilt and self-hatred at their inability to adopt the mothering role that society expects from them and that they expect from themselves.

It is, therefore, hardly surprising that women experiencing mental health–substance use problems are at greater risk of suicide than men, but some of the other risks may be less well known. Women with mental health–substance use problems are more likely to be arrested because their actions and behaviour do not reflect the accepted female stereotypes.[11] Moreover, they are at greater risk of physical illnesses, in particular obesity, diabetes and sexually transmitted diseases, than males.[10] They are more likely to be physically, emotionally and/or sexually abused.[11] Mental health–substance use is, therefore, not a particularly accurate description of the multiple health problems affecting women who have mental health–substance use problems.

ACCESSING SUPPORT

The complexity of these health needs means that these women need healthcare services that address multiple needs, including mental, physical and social, and provide care and treatment, with a non-judgemental attitude. They may also need access to housing and childcare facilities. Contemporary health services tend to compartmentalise their services: come here for mental health; go there for physical health; and there for substance use issues, and somewhere else again for housing and child care.

When asked to contribute to this chapter, both writers initially felt a little overwhelmed. Used to discussing the issues of integrated treatment for mental health–substance use problems at a broad level, also used to discussing consumer participation and its importance, it was challenging to drill down to women specifically; this took some reflection both clinically and personally. The writers did not feel they should speak on behalf of the individual; they could speak about the systems and clinical challenges in regards to women, but both felt it imperative to convey the voice of women experiencing mental health–substance use problems. So Mikah was approached to be a contributing author in this chapter.

INTRODUCING MIKAH

Mikah is an individual who is journeying along the path to recovery from mental illness–substance use problems. This is her story and her thoughts. Mikah's contribution is valued and she has had input into the chapter as a whole, as well as writing her own story. Too often in practice we forget the lived experience of the individuals we work with. Mikah's story serves as a reminder, and demonstrates the future path we as professionals need to take to ensure better services for those experiencing mental health–substance use problems.

Mikah's story

I was a package of spontaneity and compulsiveness, with rude behaviour, until I was 40 years old, due to being bipolar and a full-time drug addict (drug of choice from 27 to 40 was heroin). Between 17 and 27 I had tried all the other drugs and alcohol. It felt like a long time of being lost and mixed up.

At 17 I had to leave home because there was abuse and neglect. There was no love at home. After leaving home I held down two jobs and completed year 12. Then I went back to Detroit, where I come from, where I partied on coke and alcohol for a year. Then I returned to Melbourne and opened a record store called Spinners, for 12 months. I had super manic highs and lows all the way through these times. I knew that I had depression, so I went to lots of doctors. These doctors tried me on lots of different types of antidepressants; they only made me worse. Then I got heavier into drugs. It became a way of coping and existing. When lithium did not work, I gave doctors a miss for a while!

From my experience, it took the system until I was 38 to pick up I had more than a drug and alcohol problem to cope and deal with, I also had a mental illness. I had to endure feeling different from everybody, not understanding why I was how I was. I just thought I was weird because I heard voices, hallucinated, had suicidal thoughts and on the flip side I would imagine I was a famous DJ. I had some grandiose ideas. I used to believe I was a child of the future who had come back to learn her lessons. This resulted in some extremely self-destructive behaviour which hurt others and myself a lot. I believe pain is personal and we all cope with it differently. Sometimes I suffered anxiety or panic attacks; other times psychosis or nervous breakdowns, usually accompanied by paranoia. I often played Russian roulette, with needles, taking risks with heroin use, which was not funny.

My impulsive behaviour was often the catalyst for obtaining drugs for myself and my friends, who only used and abused me. I had violent relationships with men. I didn't know what real love was. I thought that the 'danger' of the daily chase was an adventure . . . I now know what real relationships are about. Helen Barnacle said it well in an interview she did with *Australian Story*:

> Around that time I started mixing with a group of people who were using drugs. I didn't realise it at the time but that feeling of instant gratification of when the heroin enters your bloodstream is a very momentary feeling and you don't realise it's a only a very short term solution to your worries or your emotional pain and that in fact it leads you down a path of self-destruction.[12]

In my opinion sometimes the only outcome for long-term drug addicts are prison, institutions and death, especially if they don't realise they need help.

Many times I came into contact with the law and nearly went to jail, except the magistrate would let me off because I had a mental illness.

One time at the solicitor's office where I was already in trouble I got into more trouble for stealing a wallet from the solicitor's secretary's handbag. As a result I was locked up for three days in a holding cell; this scared me a lot.

I have never been a violent offender but that day there was a lot of drama and I received a lot of attention, which I was secretly crying out for as I needed help. However, the first thing I did when they released me was go and organise a hit.

In hospital I found I had to set boundaries with my fellow inmates regarding cigarettes, phone numbers, etc.

During one of my stays at hospital I was traumatised, as were all the other 'inmates', by this man who was masturbating naked in his room with the door opened. I had to get the nurse to deal with it. For me as a woman in hospital I felt vulnerable, threatened and powerless. It reminded me of past trauma, which many women in hospital had also experienced; coping with sexual issues or confrontations in hospital made it harder to get well. When you are in hospital you feel at the mercy of staff and the behaviour of other consumers, isolated. I was glad to get home, I felt safer at home and more able to start getting well at home. Or so I hoped . . .

I was very depressed and sick of having a drug addiction and fixation. It felt like 'living on the dark side of the moon', total desperation and misery, only just surviving from day to day, sometimes hour by hour. I had hit rock bottom and wanted to end it all! So I decided to throw myself in front of a Mercedes. It was Ken's. Ken and I became instant best friends; he was absolutely straight (still is, he does not drink or smoke). Ken helped me with unconditional love, then tough love. When I was acutely ill he would always listen to my 'broken record' with one hundred per cent effort, time and support.

Later he told me he could see the gold in me; in the long run he has been proven to be right. I now have stability and security, which I did not have before.

All my so-called friends are gone as there are no drugs for them; in retrospect nearly all were broke and desperate.

I tried just about everything to quit heroin, methadone, subutex/buprenorphine, and endless times at detox[ification], at home and through drug and alcohol inpatient programmes. We are all products of our experiences and victims of circumstance, responsible for our own actions. I often have a fear of being left alone, have trouble taking care of myself and I often feel as though I am a burden to everyone else.

I am now approaching four years clean off heroin and I feel free and better at controlling my life and my state of mind. I use to be ashamed of my behaviour and how I thought. Now I 'live on the light side of the sun'. I now value myself and have constructively achieved things I am proud of. I believe alcohol and drug issues and bipolar must be treated together, because the two go hand in hand lived through by the consumer. Ultimately, I would like to see our society accept people with a mental illness (a condition), without fear or stigma attached. Then people really can be themselves. I often felt lost in the system and deprived of support and understanding, from 17 to 38. One of the most difficult things for me was to get treatment for both my bipolar disorder and my substance abuse at the same time, e.g. when I'd ring one service they would tell me to ring the other one and vice versa! As a consumer I respect and want empathy, but we loathe sympathy. I have learnt to listen to others; I no longer talk at people, but talk with them.

As of 8 November 2005 I have been off heroin. It has been a long journey but worth it.

Here are some quotes about life, which I feel are worth reading and may help others:

1 Fear knocked on the door, Faith answered, and there was no one there.[13]
2 If you live in the past, you die in the past. Live in the now and look forward to your future.[14]
3 If you can keep your head when all about you
  Are losing theirs and blaming it on you.
  If you can trust yourself when all men doubt you,
  But make allowance for their doubting too.[15]

I am starting to cultivate new friends. I work on nine different committees in mental health. I still have a fight on my hands, but I feel I am getting there and the feeling is wonderful.

CONCLUSION

Tackling the problem of mental health–substance use in women must start by understanding the experience from the individuals' perspective. As professionals, our aim is to understand the needs of the individual and how these identified needs can be addressed. Through this understanding we can work towards the development of services that provide care and treatment in a supportive and non-judgemental environment that promotes self-esteem, rather than destroying what is left of it.

REFERENCES

1 Minkoff K. Developing standards of care for individuals with co-occurring psychiatric and substance use disorders. *Psychiatric Services.* 2001; **52**: 5078–90.
2 Drake RE, Wallach MA, Alverson HS, *et al.* Psychosocial aspects of substance abuse by clients with severe mental illness. *Journal of Nervous and Mental Diseases.* 2002; **190**: 100–6.
3 Department of Human Services, Victoria. *Dual Diagnosis: key directions and priorities for service.* Melbourne: Department of Human Services, Victoria; 2007. Available at: www.health.vic.gov.au/mentalhealth/dualdiagnosis/dualdiagnosis2007.pdf (accessed 17 June 2010).
4 Judd F, Armstrong S, Kulkarni J. Gender-sensitive mental health care. *Australasian Psychiatry.* 2009; **17**: 105–11.
5 Chessler P. *Women and Madness.* New York: Four Walls Eight Windows; 1997, pp. 78–9.
6 Stewart S, Watson S, Montague R, *et al.* Set up to fail? Consumer participation in the mental health service system. *Australasian Psychiatry.* 2008; **16**: 348–53.
7 Cowan L, Deering D, Crowe M, *et al.* Alcohol and drug treatment for women: clinicians' practice. *International Journal of Mental Health Nursing.* 2003; **12**: 48–55.
8 Kelly PJ, Blacksin B, Mason E. Factors affecting substance abuse treatment completion for women. *Issues in Mental Health Nursing.* 2001; **22**: 287–304.

9 Snow D, Smith T, Branham S. Women with bipolar disorder who use alcohol and other drugs. *Journal of Addictions Nursing.* 2008; **19**: 55–60.

10 Birch S, Lavender T, Cupitt C. The physical healthcare experiences of women with mental health problems: status versus stigma. *Journal of Mental Health.* 2005; **14**: 61–72.

11 Katz-Saltzman S, Biegel DE, Townsend A. The impact of caregiver-care recipient relationship quality on family caregivers of women with substance-use disorders or co-occurring substance and mental disorders. *Journal of Family Social Work.* 2008; **11**: 141–65.

12 Barnacle H. Terms of endearment. *Australian Story.* 20 July 2000. Available at: www.abc.net.au/austory/transcripts/s152106.htm (accessed 17 June 2010).

13 Author unknown: Old English proverb.

14 Author unknown.

15 Rudyard Kipling. If. Available at: www.kipling.org.uk/kip_fra.htm (accessed 26 October 2010).

TO LEARN MORE

- Australia and New Zealand Dual Diagnosis website: www.dualdiagnosis.org.au/home/
- Victorian Dual Diagnosis resource website: www.comorbidity.org.au/
- Australian Mental Health Consumer Network: http://amhcn.org.au/
- *beyondblue* is a national, independent; not-for-profit organisation that works to address issues associated with depression, anxiety and related substance misuse disorders in Australia: www.beyondblue.org.au/

CHAPTER 5

The older adult's perspective

Wayne Skinner, Marilyn White-Campbell,
Helen MR Meier and Meldon Kahan

The aim of this chapter is to explore the interface between the lived experience of older people with mental health–substance use problems and the professionals who can identify, and respond to, these issues therapeutically. This requires a willingness to work directly not only with the older person but with others, most usually family members.

This task will be approached by reviewing processes and phases of care that people move through as issues related to their problems, from identification through engagement, preparation and active treatment through to continuing care and support. The chapter gives consideration to the issues, challenges and opportunities that apply to the initial processes of engaging older people who may be experiencing mental health–substance use problems.

Alma's story 5.1 Part I

Alma, a 74-year-old woman, was brought to the emergency department one Sunday evening. She had been a secretary for 21 years to the director of a large company, retiring nearly 10 years previously, after a career of nearly 25 years.
The middle daughter of five children, she had never married, living with her mother until her mother developed dementia and needed to be moved to a nursing home. Her mother stayed there till her death two years ago, from complications resulting from a fall. Alma has continued living in her parents' home. She has had good peer relationships with a few close women friends through her adult years, and has worked at keeping good relationships with her three nieces. One of them, Betty, has been staying with her for the past two months while she studies at a college near Alma's home. Returning earlier than expected one Sunday afternoon, Betty heard sobbing and found her aunt Alma disoriented and confused in the kitchen. There was evidence of lunch on the table, and her aunt's medication bottles, together with a brandy glass and a bottle of sherry. A calendar also lay on the table indicating it was the anniversary of Betty's mother's death, two years ago. When her aunt did not remember that Betty had been living with her, and had no recall of what had happened that day, Betty had called for paramedic help to get Alma taken to hospital.

Frank's story 5.2 Part I

Frank was one of the oldest people at the oldest methadone clinics in the country. Frank had attended since it was established in the early 1960s. Meeting a professional on the street who had also worked in the field, but not as long as Frank had been attending, the professional had been reflecting on the changes in the field over a 25-year period. When asked about the changes he had seen, Frank commented that there had been many, including the loss of many people who had died tragically of causes related to drug use because they had gone back to the street. Frank, who had struggled with depression and drug dependence all his life, now in his early 70s, had made it to old age. The professional asked Frank if he thought that being in drug treatment and receiving methadone had been factors in his longevity. Frank thought for a moment, and then admitted that, yes, it probably had. But as he turned to go, he said he sometimes wondered what life would have been like if he had been able to get away from methadone and get off drugs altogether.

REFLECTIVE PRACTICE EXERCISE 5.1

Time: 20 minutes

Take time to think about:

- Images that you have about older people and about people becoming older.
- People you know who you would consider old.
- What are the impressions that emerge?
- If you were sorting them on a ledger of negative and positive attributes, how would it look on balance?
- Are there more points on the positive side than the negative?
- When you think about your own ageing, how do you feel about getting to the point where others would consider you an old person?
- How does that feel? What does that mean for you?

AGEING AS A LIVED EXPERIENCE: BECOMING OLDER

Growing old is hard for most people. We live in a society that privileges youth, where advertising messages stigmatise and create anxiety about growing old, including 'anti-ageing' attitudes. Yet we all grow older. This in itself creates challenges to which each of us is vulnerable. This is not solely a matter of self-perception, but how we are seen, and experience ourselves being seen by others.

On the positive side of the ledger are images of wisdom, maturity and durability. Reaching retirement confers with it the prerogative and the discretion to follow personal interests rather than obligation in how one lives one's day. On the other side, there is the assumption and recognition of diminishing capability to keep up with the daily demands of work. Retirement represents an accommodation by society to those who are moving into a stage of life. With retirement, we are entering the last stage of the life journey, if we are lucky enough to have made it that far.

In terms of mental health–substance use issues, there are people who have travelled into the later part of their lives as survivors, despite the epidemiological data that suggest that most people with these problems do not survive into old age. An additional and larger population experiencing mental health–substance use problems may survive beyond 65 years.[1-3]

A further group of older people will experience these problems for the first time in their later years. This is for a variety of reasons, only some related to the socio-existential reality of being old, isolated, poor and diminished, including organic changes that lead to decline in cognitive and behavioural capacity. Others may develop substance use problems as a result of psychoactive effects of medication prescribed for medical conditions, including tolerance and psychological dependence.

Other individuals may experience alcohol, gambling and behavioural problems into which vulnerable members of the population are lured by advertising, marketing with false incentives that exploit the vulnerability associated with their loneliness and social isolation.[4]

For this stage of the journey to end well, of which death is the final destination, the challenge intensifies: maintaining ego integrity, resisting demoralisation and sustaining hope. At its best, the third age is the culmination of a process of growth and accomplishment, with a sense of succession and legacy, however modest an individual's contribution may seem. Too few people seem to see the approach of the end of their lives from this perspective. Therefore, growing old, and being an older person, can be hard.

Biological factors, including changes in health and diminishing capacities, along with psychological factors, including apprehensiveness about an unclear journey with a clear destination, social factors, for example losses such as reduced resources, and frequent bereavements make the expectable journey through old age challenging for many people. When people continue the life journey experiencing mental health–substance use issues, the challenges are even greater. It is, however, worth remembering that many people with previous experiences of mental health substance use problems may have moved beyond these problems, and are in remission. Indeed research suggests that remission is more common than not.[5] Those individuals demonstrate resilience. They also have a vulnerability that can be activated by the stresses of later life. Of more concern are the groups of individuals who have struggled with these problems in earlier years and are still striving to manage them. Finally, there is the growing number of individuals who will have late-onset mental health–substance use issues that emerge in their older years without apparent previous history.

Each of the scenarios depicted represent some of the dilemmas and challenges when mental health–substance use issues occur in the journey of later life.

REFLECTIVE PRACTICE EXERCISE 5.2

Time: 30 minutes

An older person is experiencing mental health symptoms and the negative effects of substance use behaviour.

- How much self-awareness would you expect the person to have?
- How comfortable and confident are they likely to be about acknowledging and discussing these problems with the people in their everyday lives who care about them?
- How ready might they be to approach their primary care doctor or other professional to seek help?
- How responsive do you think they will be if a spouse, a family member or a friend expresses concerns about these issues and recommends that help be sought?
- What factors might lead the family members to seek advice, if the individual refuses their suggestions and efforts to encourage direct help?
- What are the ethical dilemmas?

DISCUSSING AND EXPLORING MENTAL HEALTH–SUBSTANCE USE PROBLEMS IN OLDER PEOPLE

Where a person takes the initiative to raise concerns about their behaviour and their health, or is willing to follow the suggestions of a concerned family member or friend, the task of seeking and accepting help is already on a positive footing. However, it is often the case that the prospect of talking with a healthcare professional about behaviours that might have a substance use component, or about signs and symptoms that might indicate failing mental health, is something to avoid rather than to embrace.

It takes skill and ability to be able to work effectively in such situations where a task-oriented, question-and-answer approach is not likely to be adequate to find out what issues are really active.

It will be important to proceed in ways that are more skilfully guided by using the interpersonal process rather than formal fact-finding, assessment and diagnosis. This requires the older individual to feel safe to share information with the professional, and that the professional is actively concerned in understanding how things are, and how things stand from the point of view of the older individual. This is the case whether the individual is being seen by a professional on their own or with a concerned family member or friend.

A simple three-point model[6] for working with people experiencing mental health–substance use problems, which can be used as a grounding context for any clinical involvement, be it a single encounter, or an ongoing helping relationship, is:

1 Connect
2 Understand
3 Proceed.

These three words – **connect**, **understand**, **proceed** – may imply that this is a simple business, but there is real skill and art in the accomplishment of these essential tasks. Increasingly, there is an evidence base supporting not just the effectiveness of accomplishing these tasks, but helping us understand how to do it. That evidence suggests that if we want to be optimally effective, the 'connect' component of this model of clinical engagement is key. This is particularly important in the difficult circumstances where it will not be effective to move directly to blunt questions about mental health–substance use problems.

1 Connect

There is increasing attention placed on welcoming the person seeking assistance and care when they reach out for help. This can be on the telephone, in person and, increasingly, online. The encounter needs to be thought of, informed by and designed to address the perspective of people within/using healthcare and social services. This does not mean that the needs of the professional providing these services are unimportant or even secondary. They need to align with and complement the needs of older people, ensuring, as professionals, they provide a sense of warmth and welcome. This highlights the importance of all professionals, from the receptionist and the first contact, to the look and feel of the waiting room, the greeting on the phone and the friendliness of a website. Key considerations for engaging the individual are highlighted in Box 5.1.

BOX 5.1 Key considerations in engaging older persons

- Elder specific
- Harm reduction approach to substance use
- Use of a non-judgemental, individualised approach to address multiple issues in treatment of the individual
- Non-confrontational
- Unnecessary to admit to a mental health–substance use problem in order to access treatment
- Motivational interviewing techniques
- Gentle and unhurried pace
- Home visiting/least intrusive approach.

More important for professionally involved in first and early contact with the individual is the evidence that the quality of that contact, in interpersonal terms, is the most important determinant of whether the person will be successfully engaged and feel satisfied with the help they receive. 'Connect' is not just a preamble to getting down to work with older people, but starts out and continues to be an essential and integral part of the work – a therapeutic task at the start, and all the way through the entire experience. With a sense of connection, the professional can more directly apply themselves to the task of understanding the older person seeking help. The work of connecting will in itself provide the professional with a better sense of understanding the older person through active, respectful and reflective listening, with a view to understanding on the individual's own terms.

Motivational skills

One evidence-based and learnable skill that equips the professional to more skilfully 'connect', understand, and proceed is motivational interviewing. Motivational interviewing (*see* Book 4, Chapter 7) is a practical philosophy that sees itself as 'a

Alma's story 5.1 Part II

In the emergency room, Alma was seen fairly quickly and her physical health assessed. There were no signs of stroke for Alma's disorientation and amnesia. In fact, she was becoming more oriented and coherent as the evening went along, although she remained anxious and emotionally distressed. Further neuropsychological testing was planned. A mental health nurse met with Alma, and then with Betty, the niece, and conferred with the doctor. It was agreed that Alma would be admitted overnight. The impression of the emergency team was that alcohol combined with prescription benzodiazepines were precipitating factors in this event. Further assessment and support with the 'concurrent disorder team' was recommended. In the morning, a social worker with the team used the events of the day before as the basis for an open conversation with Alma, using motivational interviewing techniques. This led to Alma disclosing that she had experienced grief since her mother's death and had felt demoralised since her retirement. Sometimes she found that drinking privately allowed her to settle her thoughts and feelings.

way of being with the other person,[7] and also a set of skills and techniques that have demonstrated efficacy in preparing people for change and supporting them to sustain change behaviour.

The four key skills of engagement can be remembered by the anagram '**OARS**':

O   Ask **Open questions** – those that require more than a yes/no answer.

A   **Affirm** the person as deserving of respect and assistance.

R   **Reflective listening** – listen reflectively; the person you are listening to experiences you as listening empathically and as wanting to accurately understand their story.

S   **Summarise** – pull together the key points that you hear the other person saying and reflect it in order to see if the person perceives that you understand what the concerns are.

There is another guiding focus in motivational interviewing – **evoking change talk**. By helping the individual to articulate their goals, desires, needs and intentions, ideally leading to a commitment to engage in a course on action, both on their own and with support, the professional guides the individual towards desired change. This is usually the product of a process grounded in reflectively listening. For Alma, her fear was that her problems would be objectified so that she was given 'labels' that would only make her feel more hopeless and unable to be helped. Instead, the interaction left her feeling that she needed to know more about her actual health status, and that she had been letting too many things fester unexpressed. Maybe there were ways of dealing with these issues that would not require her to drink so much. She had expressed a willingness to have the social worker visit her at home to consider joining a peer support group run collaboratively by the psychogeriatric service and the concurrent disorder programme. The assessment indicated approaches that could help her with persistent feelings of low mood.

The opportunity to use motivational interviewing does not require a formal therapeutic interview.[8] There are many occasions when interactions can have motivational potential, such as occasional encounters that professionals may have with older people who are in hospital for acute care. The skilled professional will find opportunities outside of formal, scheduled contact, to have what could be called **motivational encounters**.

Frank's story 5.2 Part II

In Frank's case, a key person for him in his visits to the methadone clinic, which could vary from daily to weekly, depending on his level of stability and functioning, was the secretary. She always greeted him by name, asked how he was doing and put him at ease by including him in casual conversations about matters of general interest. The fact that his therapist spent time focusing on his goals allowed him to get help and coaching using cognitive behavioural therapy techniques for managing his persistent dysthymic mood problems. He was eventually willing to explore antidepressant medications, despite his concerns about possible side-effects, in addition to his daily methadone for opioid dependence. When situational stress caused him to relapse, he learned over time to more openly report and seek help, and talked about strategies to avoid relapse by recognising stress and other triggers. He especially appreciates the recognition by professionals that, as he gets older, he has mobility problems – coming to the clinic requires a 45-minute bus ride across town and he can access his methadone from a local pharmacy, checking by telephone on an as-needed basis. The clinic proposed to transfer his care to his family doctor, but Frank wants to be sure that he is somewhere where his complex issues can be understood and addressed.

2 Understand

The process of connecting through the use of the OARS skills are to be found in similar format in humanistic counselling approaches across all bio-medical and psychosocial professions and disciplines. This sets the stage for understanding, which is the necessary antecedent for determining how to proceed. The key here is that understanding is not a unilateral or one-sided task. It is a mutual process that acknowledges the individual's right and need to understand, as well as the professional's need and requirement to make a formulation of what issues the individual is experiencing. It includes the active and positive role of family and friends who are willing to play a part in whatever processes of care are needed to help the older person achieve the best possible levels of well-being and functioning. For too many people, access to social support is not optimal. But in many cases, even with limitations, there are possibilities. Both Frank and Alma, for example, have some social support that they can mobilise, although it could be enhanced.

Understanding is a process that continues. It is a growing body of information that applies to the specific situation that is being addressed. For the individual, it includes not only information about health issues and the options for addressing them, but also involvement in learning about the attitudes that professionals have towards them in the context of these physical and mental health–substance use issues. It is not merely knowing what is available but how they will be treated, welcomed, respected and included in their care. Family members will also be developing their own understanding, not only of the nature of the individual's problems but what care is available, and how they – the family – are viewed as that process develops and unfolds. Some 'Psychiatric tips' are presented in Box 5.2.

BOX 5.2 Psychiatric tips: diagnosis is the first step to care and treatment

What brings the older person to attention?
- Concurrent and coexisting mental illness and substance use interacting?
- Common factors?

What do we attend to?
- Current biological, psychological and social factors
- Current living arrangements
- Older person's strengths

What is the older person's current life experience?
- Presence of shame: individual, family, social/cultural group
- Presence of stigma: individual, family, social/cultural group
- Isolation/inclusion?

What is the older person's life story?
- Past and current medical history: head injury?
- Past and present psychiatric history: trauma?
- Past and present medication history?

Who else may know?
- Collateral history: past and present
- Collusion/complicity in substance use
- Cultural context: consider mutual assumptions about role of culture for individual
- Mutually understood language: important to have interpreter, not informant
- Confidentiality and information gathering
- Disclosure requires consent
- Information may be received from collateral sources
- Information seeking continues throughout encounters
- Information gathering may be therapeutic: life review.

For the professional, there are a number of key dimensions creating a matrix within which a comprehensive understanding of the problems and solutions for the older person can be constructive. There are four main elements that can be remembered by the mnemonic '**SCIO**', which is, aptly enough, the Latin verb meaning 'to know'.

1 **Subjective** factors refer to the information and perspectives the person makes available to us as they share their lived experience of the issues that are of concern. So much of what we have to go on in mental health–substance use comes from the self-report of the individual, in this case the older person, who we are attempting to help. This reinforces the merits of connecting – using the helping relationship – to encourage the individual to engage using the resources and services available to them.

2 **Collateral** sources can be invaluable in developing effective understanding of older people who may experience mental health–substance use problems. Even when the expert evaluation of a person's health status in the moment is precise, it leaves unanswered the longitudinal, lifespan context, which can be so often fathomed by input from others who have known the person for some time. Consent is required to provide others with information about the individual's health status and other psychosocial information, but it is not required to listen to others who want to share information, or to answer questions that may be beneficial towards forming effective understanding of the individual. Collateral information can also include formal sources, such as other professionals and service systems – criminal justice, social services, and community affiliations – faith groups and churches.

3 **Impressionistic** knowledge that we, as professionals, form through the opportunity to observe and interact with individuals. This knowledge is informed by observation and by conceptual and theoretical perspectives on human behaviour, functioning and development. Moreover, it is informed by the practical wisdom derived from knowledge gained by working with individuals who have experienced mental health–substance use problems. Bringing that to bear and adding the other vectors of knowledge enhances understanding of problems and solutions in ways that can be focused and person-centred.

4 **Objective** knowledge is a growing domain of clinical acumen. This includes anything from lab tests that provide information through blood work and urinalysis to CT scans and MRIs to psychological tests that help screen and assess the presence of mental health–substance use problems.

The understanding that can be potentially brought to bear is formidable. It is a building process that takes time and active involvement. No one vector of knowledge is adequate for effective action in the treatment of these problems. Each has a vital role to play in the engagement of older people in processes of care that provide the services and support which produce better responses, from the perspective of the individual, family and professional.

3 Proceed

While connecting and understanding are intrinsically important tasks in any collaborative approach to therapy, the intended goal is to be helpful. These create an enhanced possibility that the professional, the family and the individual can proceed to the best course of action. This course is shaped by the stage of the helping process for which we are concerned. In this chapter, that stage is the initial stage of engagement. As that succeeds the stages of preparation, followed by active treatment and continuing care, develop and emerge, depending on the effectiveness of the work to date.

At the level of engagement, there are some formal tools that can be used for screening for the presence of mental health–substance use problems. But the focus here is not on individuals with active and healthy social support, who confidently and with commitment seek expert help to attend to problems they themselves recognise and desire to change. The exploration of these issues will in most cases be careful, tentative and gradual. For example, the MAST-G[9] – a version of the MAST screener for alcohol problems for older people – has been found by some to be more sensitive to identifying alcohol problems than a four-question screener called the CAGE,[10] which is frequently promoted in the literature on screening and brief intervention. Yet there will be many cases where the professional might, because of circumstances, be able to ask only one question. Current advice is to ask: 'Have you had five or more standard drinks of alcohol on any one occasion in the past month?' However, the professional might want to ask more openly, 'Have you had any concerns about your drinking?' followed by 'Has anyone else ever expressed concern to you about your drinking?'

These tentative strategies may be more appropriate where relationships are not yet formed and apprehensiveness and fear are high. As connection and understanding grow, candour – a mutual trait in any good relationship, therapeutic ones included – becomes more possible.

KEY POINT 5.1

Engagement is the primary focus. EM Forster's two word epigram for his novel *Howard's End* is: 'Only connect.' In working motivationally, our goal is: 'Always connect!'

For purposes stated here, engagement is the primary focus. It is important to recognise the multiple dimensions that the problems and needs of older people experiencing mental health–substance use problems can involve. This multiplicity can occur in the context of acuity (the hot issues that bring immediacy to the need for a helping response) or in the context of chronicity (recurrent and persistent issues, with varying degrees of severity, which impinge on the person's life). The other aspect is complexity: this is not a single vector of illness, but the co-occurrence of at least two significant problem areas. Not only that, but these problems can have acute and chronic intersections with physical health and with social problems. They need to be understood and addressed from a diversity framework that includes consideration of race, gender, culture and class and – increasingly as the social demographic in the global community changes – age and the problems of ageing.

The family physician (general practitioner) has an important role in the ongoing care of the individual and family. Continued drinking, for example, may be used to avoid withdrawal symptoms, which tend to be more prolonged and severe than in younger adults. The physician can organise a medical detoxification in the home or clinic; this will prevent the medical complications of unplanned and untreated withdrawal. Table 5.1 offers an illustration of the physician's role in managing substance use problems.

TABLE 5.1 Family physician's role in managing and addressing mental health–substance use problems in the older adult

Role	Example	Comment
Identification	Alcohol history Screening questionnaire (CAGE,[10] AUDIT[11]) Laboratory: gamma-glutamyltransferase (GGT), mean corpuscular volume (MCV)	Alcohol history and screening questionnaires have sensitivity of 70%–80% in primary care settings. Laboratory tests useful for confirming clinical suspicion and monitoring progress in treatment.
Planned treatment of alcohol withdrawal	Office or home Lorazepam every 1–2 hours until symptoms resolved (*see* Toolkit for full protocol)	The older adult has more prolonged and severe withdrawal and is more likely to develop complications, such as delirium. Symptom-triggered benzodiazepine treatment shortens length of stay and reduces rates of delirium and seizures.
Pharmacotherapy	Examples: disulfiram, naltrexone, acamprosate, topiramate	Pharmacotherapy can improve drinking outcomes. These medications reduce craving and reinforcing effects of alcohol. Disulfiram causes sickness when alcohol consumed; effective when dispensed by a family member. Close monitoring is essential when using disulfiram as it can be fatal if taken with alcohol.
Counselling	Brief advice, repeated each office or home visit	Brief counselling interventions by physicians have been shown to be effective at reducing alcohol use in the older adult. Older people are more likely than younger people to see an alcohol counsellor when referred from a healthcare setting.
Safe prescribing of medications	Benzodiazepine tapering	Benzodiazepine use in the older adult is associated with falls, worsening of mood, and cognitive impairment. Safe, effective protocols exist for benzodiazepine tapering.
Medical complications, e.g. liver cirrhosis	Education Diet (low sodium and protein) Medications (e.g. beta-blockers)	Medical care can prevent complications of cirrhosis, encephalopathy, ascites, bleeding oesophageal varices.

(*continued*)

Role	Example	Comment
Psychiatric comorbidity	Diagnosis and treatment of depression and alcohol dependence	Antidepressant therapy and counselling can help decrease drinking and increase mood. Access to alcohol treatment is a protective factor for suicide in the older adult.
Cognitive impairment	Diagnosis of cognitive impairment	While mild to moderate alcohol use may protect against vascular dementia, heavy alcohol use is associated with cognitive impairment in the elderly. Alcohol-dependent individuals perform worse than controls on cognitive testing, but better than individuals with Alzheimer's. Alcohol-induced cognitive impairment may improve with abstinence. Reduce the risk of Korsakoff's syndrome in heavy drinking by giving vitamin B_1 regularly by injection (orally may have poor absorption); abstinence can improve memory in people experiencing Korsakoff's psychosis.

Alma's story 5.1 Part III

The social worker visited Alma at home, post-discharge. Alma did have the perception that the professionals were working as a team. She could rely on any of them to be up to date in terms of what was happening with her. The team wanted to build more social support for Alma, including more family and peer connection. This was not an easy thing for Alma, given her inclination to try to manage on her own and her difficulty in feeling comfortable in many informal social situations. She did find that the prescribed medication seemed to lessen her panic. She had also found it helpful to join a peer social support group where others her age, with whom she could identify, were getting together to talk about similar challenges in their lives. As her sense of personal well-being increased, she expressed an interest in having some sort of volunteer role. She offered to use her secretarial and organisational skills to work with others who want to set up an advocacy and information service for older people in her community.

Frank's story 5.2 Part III

Frank survived into old age, despite serious problems that could have affected his longevity. Eventually, he did have health problems that have required him to seek more medical support. A lifelong tobacco smoker, he was diagnosed with emphysema. He had very little motivation to discontinue smoking, but approached his illness and decline usually with good humour and even gratitude, although not without irritability and stress at times. He was able to adjust to changes in care that were more oriented to physical health management, including the need for oxygen. He was worried if being on methadone would compromise the care he would receive for any pain that might accompany his declining health. The good knowledge base and working alliance he had with the professionals has made it productive to raise health concerns and to find solutions that mattered to him.

REFLECTIVE PRACTICE EXERCISE 5.3

Time: 30 minutes
- How credible are these narratives?
- Against a background of many stories of failed engagement, is it possible to imagine and to begin to insist that these processes be better, so that older people who need care for often complex problems can get the care and assistance that is needed?
- Which ways already in use demonstrate a 'connect-understand-proceed' logic for clinical engagement?
- In which ways can you use interactive occasions with the older person and their family to produce motivational encounters?
- How does working together help to move towards the next stages of preparation, active change and continuing care?

CONCLUSION

Consideration of the perspective of older adults includes attention to the interface between their lived experience and the frame of reference of the professionals working to assess them and offer them care. Members of a team individually and collectively require an approach that includes and involves the others important in the life of an older adult, usually family but also community workers and informal caregivers. Processes and phases of care for an older adult progress from identification of issues to engagement, with preparation for and initiation of active treatment, followed by continuing care and support in the person's own context.

Issues, challenges and opportunities arise during each phase of care, in particular the initial processes of engaging an older adult who is identified with concurrent disorders, with attention to efforts to understand the determinants of the mental health and substance use problems.

In summary, this chapter outlines an approach which starts with skilfully working to connect with an older adult, then to understand the person's perspective in terms of life context (with its past, present and future aspects), as well as capacity for consent and participation. Those tasks done, professional and individual proceed based on collaborative planning, with action steps that ideally involve family, peers and a circle of social support in an environment with facilitative resources and services. Usually, the realities of a particular individual's circumstances do not fit such an ideal formula for effective care. The skill in helping involves a pragmatic talent for artfully mobilising a plan of care that draws on positive factors in suboptimal circumstances, guided by an ability to negotiate the difference between the ways things ought to be and the way they are.

REFERENCES

1 Haver B, Giestad R, Lindberg S, *et al.* Mortality risk up to 25 years after initiation of treatment among 420 Swedish women with alcohol addiction. *Addiction.* 2009; **104**: 413–19.

2 Miller N. Mortality risks in alcoholism and effects of abstinence and addiction treatment. *Psychiatric Clinics of North America.* 1999; **22**: 371–83.

3 Goldbloom DS, Kurdyak P. Mental illness and cardiovascular mortality: searching for the links. *Canadian Medical Association Journal.* 2007; **13**(176): 787–8.

4 Alexander B. *The Globalization of Addiction: a study in poverty of the spirit.* Oxford: Oxford University Press; 2007.

5 Heyman GM. *Addiction: a disorder of choice.* Cambridge, MA: Harvard University Press; 2009.

6 Skinner WJW, editor. *Treating Concurrent Disorders: a guide for counsellors.* Toronto, ON: Centre for Addiction and Mental Health; 2005.

7 Miller WR, Rollnick S. *Motivational Interviewing: preparing people for change.* 2nd ed. New York: Guilford; 2002.

8 Rollnick S, Miller WR, Butler CC. *Motivational Interviewing in Health Care: helping patients change behavior.* New York: Guilford Press; 2008.

9 Blow FC, Brower KJ, Schulenberg JE, *et al.* The Michigan Alcoholism Screening Test – Geriatric Version (MAST-G): a new elderly-specific screening instrument. *Alcoholism: Clinical and Experimental Research.* 1992; **16**: 372.

10 Mayfield D, McLeod G, Hall P. The CAGE questionnaire: validation of a new alcoholism screening instrument. *American Journal of Psychiatry.* 1974; **131**: 1121–3.

11 Babor TF, Higgins-Biddle JC, Saunders JB, *et al.* *The Alcohol Use Disorders Identification Test: guidelines for use in primary care.* 2nd ed. Geneva: World Health Organization; 2001. Available at: http://whqlibdoc.who.int/hq/2001/who_msd_msb_01.6a.pdf (accessed 19 July 2010).

TO LEARN MORE

- CAMH Healthy Ageing Project. *Improving Our Response to Older Adults with Substance Use, Mental Health and Gambling Problems: a guide for supervisors, managers and clinical staff.* Toronto: Centre for Addiction and Mental Health; 2008. www.camh.net/Publications/Resources_for_Professionals/Improving_Our_Response/camh_healthy_aging_project.html

- Primary Care Addiction Toolkit. CAMH Knowledge Exchange. http://knowledgex.camh.net/primary_care/toolkits/addiction_toolkit/Pages/default.aspx

- O'Grady C, Skinner WJW. *A Family Guide to Concurrent Disorders.* Toronto: Centre for Addiction and Mental Health; 2007. www.camh.net/publications/resources_for_professionals/partnering_with_families/partnering_families_famguide.pdf

- Seniors' Mental Health and Substance Use Issue. HereToHelp Information You Can Trust. BC Partners for Mental Health and Addictions Information; 2009. www.heretohelp.bc.ca/publications/factsheets/seniors

- Centre for Substance Abuse Treatment. TIP 26: Substance Abuse among Older Adults. *SAMHSA/CSAT Treatment Improvement Protocols.* Rockville, MD: Substance Abuse and Mental health Services Administration; 1998. www.ncbi.nlm.nih.gov/book/NBK14467/

CHAPTER 6

The young person's perspective

Ilana B Crome and Alexander Baldacchino

CHAPTER LEARNING OBJECTIVES

To understand that:

➤ young people have the highest risk of substance use across the life course
➤ young people presenting for treatment often have multiple needs
➤ risk factors are complex and interactive: findings are most consistent for the influence of family
➤ a developmental perspective takes account of the impact of different stages on the initiation, continuation or cessation of mental health–substance use
➤ clinical presentation in young people may differ from adults
➤ intervention involves early detection and early intervention and a degree of assertiveness in follow-up
➤ policy is heavily focused on young people and families, but an understanding of the mechanisms that underpin the development of mental health–substance use conditions in young people is in its infancy.

Adolescents receiving treatment for substance problems are more likely to have multiple drug problems as well as emotional and behavioural problems and to report poorer health than those who do not receive treatment.[1] Although young people who are at risk of poor health outcomes are least likely to approach services, they may present in some form to all the major specialties in medical and social work practice. Even if the individual presents with a substance problem, this may not be his or her major problem; conversely, the presenting problem may not be immediately recognised as relating to substance use.[2] Taking account of the stage of development at time of presentation is key to understanding how mental health–substance use has evolved, and how it should be treated.

COMORBID CONDITIONS IN THE YOUNGER POPULATION

In general terms, this period of life confers the highest risk for the development of substance use disorders and psychological problems, and those with the most severe substance disorders are likely to suffer psychiatric and physical health disorders as well as substance use problems.[3] However, even though there may be a reduction of substance use during adulthood, the consequences may linger on as it is estimated that about 90% of adults who are dependent started to use during adolescence, and half initiated substance use before the age of 15. Early onset of substance use is related to a higher rate of dependence and mental illness. About 80% of people entering substance use treatment experience a mental illness.[4]

Illicit drug use

Sixteen to 24-year-olds form one-sixth of the English and Welsh population. Young people generally report higher levels of drug use than older people. Adolescents may become dependent much more quickly than do adults and overall mortality of adolescent addicts is 16 times that of the general adolescent population. The latest data from the UK National Health Service Information Centre on 11- to 15-year-olds has demonstrated a fall in those who have tried drugs at least once, from 29% in 2001 to 25% in 2007, but 10% (300 000) were likely to have taken drugs in the past week.[5] People aged 20–24 use approximately twice as many illicit drugs as 16- to 19-year-olds. Class A drug use among young people has remained stable since 1998 and the reported use of any drug in the previous year actually fell in the 16–29 age groups between 1998 and 2006/7. Over the course of their lifetime, 2.75 million (44.7%) young people aged 16–24 had used an illicit drug, 1.5 million (24%) had used an illicit drug in the previous year, and 1 million (14.3%) in the previous month. One million (16.3%) had used a Class A drug during their lifetime, 500 000 (8.1%) in the previous year and 250 000 (4.3%) in the previous month. Young women are one and a half to three times more likely to use substances than older women.[6] International studies demonstrate that about one quarter to one-fifth of women in younger age groups have used illicit drugs in the past year.

Alcohol

In comparison to other countries, UK consumption of alcohol is rising, especially in women and young people. When considering the overall population impact, it is quantity of alcohol and pattern of drinking, as well as the harm accrued and the development of dependence, that need to be taken into account. 'Binge drinking' in young people has become a particular source of concern in some countries. Although it is postulated that this behaviour does not necessarily persist into adult life, there are concerns that harms accrued during this period may be damaging in the long term. There is considerable interest around the 'risk' of harm; for example, heavy alcohol intake may lead to cirrhosis, but 'moderate' consumption may reduce the risk of coronary artery disease.

Younger drinkers are more likely to suffer accidents, assaults and acute intoxication.[7] It is estimated that 30 000 hospital admissions per year are due to alcohol dependence syndrome, and 150 000 are related to alcohol use, whereas 20 000 alcohol users die prematurely. At a conservative estimate, this costs the UK National Health Service £1.9 billion, and this excludes the inestimable cost to families and communities, partly due to alcohol-related crime and public order offences. In this context, there are 1.2 million incidents of alcohol-related violence, 80 000 arrests for drunk and disorderly behaviour, 360 000 arrests for domestic violence, and 80 000 drink-driving cases per year. These crimes include fatalities (approximately 500) and 17 000 injuries. The cost is calculated at £7.3 billion, and the emotional cost is inestimable. Unemployment and decreased productivity are additional consequences and costs. The wider, and more difficult to quantify, social harms cannot be ignored. Family relationships, stability and income diminish, with an estimated 1 million children affected by alcohol use in the family. Alcohol dependence is associated with homelessness and 'rough sleepers'.

Smoking

Teenagers who smoke appear to come more from disadvantaged backgrounds with poor educational attainment and social difficulties when experimentation commences between the ages of 11 and 13 years.[8] In the UK 20% of 11- to 16-year-olds smoked regularly, with more girls now smoking than boys.[9] Despite the overall decline in smoking over the last three decades in the UK, cigarette smoking is highest in the age group 20- to 24-year-olds. It is estimated that 38% of males and 35% of females in this age group are smokers.[10]

Young people who smoke have a higher risk of developing dependence and achieve dependence at lower smoking rates than adults, which results in a lower probability of quitting smoking in adulthood.[11-14]

As in other addictive processes there are biological (genetic, gender, age, ethnicity), behavioural or attitudinal (attitudes to substance use, religious affinity, educational aspiration), interpersonal (family relationships and friends), and environmental and economic factors (socioeconomic status, neighbourhood unrest). Mental health problems (e.g. depression and anxiety, impulsivity and sensation seeking, attention deficit hyperactivity disorder, eating disorders and other substance use) also increase the risk of smoking.[15,16]

Comorbid smoking, alcohol and other drug problems

Young people who smoke tobacco are more likely to use alcohol and illicit drugs,[17] which may manifest as problems at school, deviant behaviour and violence.[18,19] It has been noted that '*it is common to drink and not smoke, it very unusual to smoke and not drink*'.[18]

One study reviewed the relationship between cigarette smoking, other substance use and psychiatric problems.[20] In those who attend specialist services about 75% of adolescents have an additional psychiatric illness and many also suffer physical ill health. Heavier smokers were more likely to report respiratory problems, indicating the rapidity with which health problems emerge.

Depressive disorder and disruptive behaviour are consistently reported in teenage smokers.[21] Clinical samples of adolescents treated for substance use smoked more than the general population: 85% reported current smoking behaviour, 75% were daily smokers and 60% smoked 10 or more cigarettes daily.[21]

Comorbid mental health problems

It is not easy to identify the prevalence of substance use and serious mental illness in this age group since few studies focus on teenagers only. Each of the disorders may be explored, but rarely are they combined and when combined disorders are discussed the focus is not on the under-19-year-olds. The systematic review of coexistent substance use in psychosis pointed to wide variations.[23] Most recent UK studies reported rates of 20%–37% in mental health settings and 6%–15% in addiction settings. Individual, crisis and forensic settings are, not surprisingly, higher, i.e. 38%–50%. Inner cities and some ethnic groups are overrepresented. It should be emphasised that there are varying age ranges in the studies described on first episode psychosis above.

One national mental health survey study on young people aged 13–15 years old confirmed that having a psychiatric disorder was associated with substance use, and that use of one substance increased the risk of other substance being used. Interestingly, and in keeping with studies described above, these links were primarily accounted for by smoking cigarettes.[24] However, psychiatric disorders were not separately analysed and substance use was self-reported.

RISK FACTORS

There are a host of 'reasons' why people use substances, and which factors, or what interaction of factors, may influence their decisions. These may include increasing availability, low price, promotion of drinks aimed at a particular group, peer pressure, a culture which encourages 'drinking to get drunk', early onset of drinking, parental divorce, poor parental supervision, parental drinking, age, sex, region of the country, genetic predisposition and personality type. Associations or correlations between some of these so-called risk factors do not equate to causality, so that decreasing or eliminating one or more should not result in the expected reduction.[25–28]

There is a substantial epidemiological literature on factors associated with increased risk of illicit drug use among young people.[25] The nature of the evidence is complex with high-risk groups identified, such as the homeless, those looked after by local authorities, prostitutes, truants, those excluded from school, young offenders, children from families with substance misusing parents or siblings and young people with conduct or depressive disorder.

The detailed review further explored these issues and identified some inconsistencies as follows:[25]

➤ The strongest and most consistent evidence links family interaction to drug use. The key elements of family interaction are parental discipline, family cohesion and parental monitoring. Modification of parental monitoring may be effective in reducing adolescent drug use. Some aspects of family structure are linked to adolescent drug use. There is also consistent evidence linking peer drug use and drug availability to adolescent drug use. These factors probably explain the consistent findings that age is strongly associated with prevalence of drug use. There is also limited evidence linking self-esteem and hedonism to drug use. Categories where evidence linking specific factors to drug use is mixed include gender, mental health, parental substance use, attention deficit hyperactivity disorder, stimulant therapy, religious involvement, sport, health educator-led interventions, school performance, early onset of substance use, and socioeconomic status. No evidence was found linking adolescent drug use in the UK to ethnicity, language or place of birth. This does not mean that such a link does not exist, only that the review did not consider any relevant studies.

➤ The evidence points to associations between a diverse group of risk factors for drug use. These factors include parental discipline, family cohesion, parental monitoring, peer drug use, drug availability, genetic profile, self-esteem, hedonistic attitudes, reasons for drug use, and the ratio of risk:protective factors. There is less consistent evidence linking drug use to mental health, parental substance use, attention deficit hyperactivity disorder/stimulant therapy, religious involvement, sport, health educator-led interventions, school performance, early onset of substance use, and socioeconomic status.

➤ Where the causal nature of these associations has been tested in intervention trials, effects have generally been small. This could be because the factors are not readily amenable to intervention, because the associations are not causal, because the influence of individual factors is small, because finding in one population is not generalisable to others or for a combination of these reasons.

➤ Risk factors have differential predictive values throughout adolescence. Some factors may occur at birth (or before) while others occur at varying times throughout adolescence. Some factors may persist for long periods of time while others are transitory. Different factors may be associated with the initiation and continuation of drug use, although this distinction is not always clear in the literature. Risk factors are not discrete entities and their complex interactions are difficult to conceptualise, let alone analyse. The studies reviewed here indicate additive effects of risk factors (although there may also be complex interactions). The distinction between early and late-onset risk factors is important as preventive measures need to focus on particular age groups.

➤ The psychosocial developmental stage and associated cognitive, social and biological risk factors may both influence the development of mental health–substance use and the way it is manifest in a clinical situation. For example, impulsivity may feature prominently since decision-making and appreciation of risk may have not developed. The balance needs to be between supervision and the wish for independence and autonomy.

SCREENING AND ASSESSMENT

A cornerstone of treatment intervention is assessment of the nature and extent of substance use and mental health issues in the young person, so that problems can be recognised and support provided. Substance use (or misuse) is rarely a 'stand alone' issue – it tends to come embedded in a social matrix, which requires a coordinated response. Assessment can be a protracted process in young people for a variety of reasons. While in principle the objectives may appear similar to adults, professionals have to often use ingenuity and patience to engage and retain a young person long enough so that an assessment of safety and security can be undertaken in the first instance. The next key goal is to be certain that the person will return for treatment and further assessment.

Assessment and the relationship to intervention

This general protocol is adapted from one developed for nicotine dependence and is a useful way to formulate the assessment process because it translates into specific management plans.[29]

Phase 1: Ask

➤ Ask all individuals about all substance use. This should include over-the-counter medications, prescribed medications and street drugs, as well as medications shared with family members.

➤ Differentiate between substance use, abuse, harmful use and dependence. However, young people may not yet have developed a dependence, and can have very serious physical and psychosocial difficulties associated with substance use. They may differ from adults in that they have shorter duration of use, different pattern of use (e.g. bingeing), greater combinations of substances (e.g. poly-substance use), fewer or less serious medical complications, and less withdrawal and dependence features.

➤ Conceptualise assessment as ongoing. This is all the more tricky in young people with mental health–substance use problems because they may not feel well and are therefore little motivated to return.

➤ Record the information since presentations may change quickly and unpredictably.

➤ Be aware of, and sensitive to, the ambivalence substance-using individuals may feel. They are rightly concerned about confidentiality, and consent issues need to be considered.

➤ Be non-judgemental and act in a non-confrontational way, since this can be a powerful determinant of both the extent to which relevant information is elicited and engagement with the therapeutic process.

➤ Assess social (family disharmony, financial) and psychological (for positive effects or to relieve withdrawal) risk and reasons why young people may be experiencing problems.

Phase 2: Assess

➤ Assess the extent and nature of use, as well as degree of dependence for each substance.

➤ Educate individuals, family and carers about the psychological and the physical effects of substances.

➤ Inform individuals, family and carers about the relationship of withdrawal symptoms to mental and physical states.

➤ Make some assessment of the level of motivation or 'stage of change' (*see* Book 4, Chapters 6 and 7) at which the individual may be. Young people report lower stage of readiness to change. In young people this can change unpredictably.

➤ Suggest what the 'goals' may be for a particular individual at a particular stage (e.g. abstinence or harm reduction).

➤ Negotiate treatment choices and appropriateness (e.g. pharmacological interventions, the need for referral or admission to specialist services).

➤ Clinical manifestations of the condition may impair the history-taking process (e.g. lack of concentration, anxiety, depression, neurocognitive dysfunction).

➤ Follow an assessment schedule.

Phase 3: Advise

➤ Continue the assessment within a brief 5–10-minute 'motivational interviewing' framework (*see* Book 4, Chapter 7).

➤ Provide the young person with the opportunity to express their anxieties and concerns.

➤ Offer personalised feedback about clinical findings, including physical examination and laboratory tests.

➤ Outline and discuss the personal benefits and risks of continued substance use (e.g. drinking and 'safe' levels of drinking).

➤ Provide self-help materials (e.g. manuals).

Phase 4: Assist

➤ Provide support and positive expectations of success. Young people may have low self-esteem, a history of rejection, depression and anxiety.

➤ Acknowledge loss of confidence and self-esteem as a result of failed attempts.

➤ Suggest that, if the goal is abstinence, a 'quit date' be set, so that the individual can plan accordingly (e.g. get rid of any alcohol or drugs in the house) and safely (is it safe to stop drinking abruptly or not?).

➤ Work through a range of alternative coping strategies, including the identification of cues that might help distract the individual. Use techniques that are developmentally and cognitively appropriate.

Phase 5: Arrange

➤ Individual treatment for young people with mental health–substance use problems is more difficult to arrange than for adults. However, it may be necessary to refer or organise admission to a specialist or an appropriate unit, e.g. child and adolescent psychiatry services, paediatric unit, adult substance use service, if the individual:
— is in severe withdrawal, or is likely to develop severe withdrawal, including delirium tremens
— has serious medical problems related to heavy substance use
— is in unstable social circumstances (e.g. homelessness or unsuitably accommodated; subject to victimisation or abuse)
— is severely dependent on one substance or using multiple substances
— has a severe comorbid physical and/or psychiatric illness, including suicidal ideation[30,31]
— has a history of frequent relapse.

OUTCOME IN YOUNG PEOPLE

As treatment research is limited in this vulnerable group, there are many unanswered questions around what the appropriate goals and outcomes are for adolescents. As many normally functioning young people are using substances, abstinence may not be perceived as appropriate by individuals, families and professionals.[32] There is recognition that the situation is dynamic for all parties, and relapse is to be averted.[33]

The lack of treatment facilities for mental health problems in adolescents admitted for treatment of substance use disorders in the US was recently highlighted.[34] This study reviewed admission and follow-up reports on a cohort of 1088 young patients aged between 12 and 19 who were admitted to seven treatment programmes. The results indicated high levels of mental health problems at admission and at three-month follow-up. Few of those with mental health problems had received treatment for these symptoms during their drug treatment.

The importance of detection and treatment of mental health–substance use disorders in adolescents is demonstrated in the findings of a cross-sectional study of attempted suicide in 503 adolescent patients with a substance use diagnosis.[35] The risk of attempted suicide was shown to be increased when adolescents had a mood disorder in addition to their substance use disorder.

Outcome research in young people shows that, while only a small minority will achieve and maintain abstinence at one to four years after treatment, about two-thirds reduce substance use and improve in other areas, such as offending, education and employment as a result of improved confidence, self-esteem, academic attainment, mental health and family relationships.[36,37]

So, while young adults (the 18- to 25-year-old age group) have the highest rates of mental health and substance use, they are least likely to remain engaged in a treatment programme.[38,39] Damage accrued may affect the ability to reach certain milestones with long-lasting ramifications.

Evidence for effective treatment is mainly from the US, where there is emphasis on brief motivational work, cognitive behavioural therapy and multi-systemic therapies.[40,41] In the UK, there is also emphasis on harm reduction (*see* Chapter 15), including needle exchange, prevention of drug-related deaths and treatment for physical illness and injury. There is little provision or evidence for residential treatment, but it may be needed for those with chronic, relapsing states.

The involvement of the family may be necessary for consent for treatment, and generally desirable for support, information and advice. Recent studies that focus on the effectiveness of active support for families and developing social skills and competence in parents and children are of relevance. The Iowa Strengthening Families Program[42] and Preparing for the Drug Free Years[43] and Community Reinforcement and Family Training (CRAFT)[44] are examples. These programmes are introduced before substance use has commenced and should promote positive parenting by raising parental awareness regarding the child's needs, supporting joint activities between parent and child, enhancing educational opportunities and care facilities for children, acting as a catalyst to encourage supervision by parents, and identifying high-risk children so that help is available for parents.

There is growing recognition that treatment has to be considered in the long term, as recovery is longer for people who started under the age of 21 and for those in high mental distress.[4] In relation to treatment for drug use, one study reported that the risk:protection ratio is a consistent predictor of the level of drug use during and after treatment.[45]

One of the first studies to confirm the negative impact of mental health–substance use on response to treatment indicates that adolescents with high levels of psychiatric mental health–substance use have high levels of dysfunction and consequently present a more difficult treatment challenge.[46] Relapse during treatment in adolescents with cannabis dependence has also been shown to be higher when there is associated coexistent depressive illness.[47] Similarly, those adolescents with alcohol use disorder and concurrent major depression have been demonstrated to relapse more quickly (survival time of 19 days to first drink) than those without (45 days to first drink). This difference was significant.[33]

One study on the impact of substance use at one year in first episode psychosis indicated a 43% baseline rate of substance use which decreased to 22% at one year.[48] Although the age range was 18–64, people with substance use at baseline were more likely to be younger, male and depressed. There were no differences in outcome in those who had never used substances and those who stopped using substances, but people who persistently used substances had more severe depression, more positive symptoms, poorer functional outcome and greater rates of relapse at one year. An Australian study reported that in a 15- to 30-year-old age group (mean age 21.6 years) substance use (53% at follow-up) was an independent risk factor for problematic recovery in first episode psychosis,[49] e.g. increased risk of admission, relapse of positive symptoms and shorter time to relapse. However, surprisingly, substance use was not associated with longer time to remission. Moreover, another study has pointed to a bidirectional relationship between substance use and cannabis relapse, in that a higher frequency of cannabis use was predictive of psychotic relapse (if medication adherence, other substance use and duration of untreated psychosis were controlled for), while an increase in psychotic symptoms was predictive of relapse to cannabis use.[50] In this study only 15% of individuals had not used any illicit substance in the previous 12 months.

A multicentre international trial has reported on the acute response to olanzapine and haloperidol in first episode schizophrenia-related psychosis and substance use.[51] Not only were first episode patients likely to have associated substance use disorder, but the presence of these disorders may influence negative responses to anti-psychotic medications – both typical and atypical – in the first 12 weeks of treatment.

At four years after treatment, 80% of those who smoked at the time of treatment were still smokers, although rates did reduce following treatment.[20] Non-smoking was related to lower rates of substance use.[52] The authors concluded that adolescents in treatment for substance use are heavy smokers and that this persists after treatment.[20] This is not because adolescents do not want to stop: two-thirds had attempted to quit, but 70% started smoking within a month of stopping.[53] These findings emphasise the need for smoking interventions that take account of the developmental needs of young people, peer influences, the development of dependence at lower levels of use than adults, and the perception of the health problems associated with cigarettes in comparison with other substances.

Key elements which contribute to quality and effectiveness of young people's services are having a comprehensive assessment, an integrated approach, family involvement, developmental appropriateness, engagement and retention, qualified staff, gender and cultural competence and evaluation of outcomes.[54] Of note was the finding that treatment quality was significantly greater in programmes offering intensive levels of care. This is relevant since mental illness makes the likelihood of relapse greater even after remission.[55]

CONCLUSION

Young people experiencing mental health–substance use problems are underserved. It is difficult to base treatment and policy on relevant research evidence. Research has to be at the core of any initiative. Some degree of substance use and mental health–substance use in young people is to be expected. Many of the factors that predispose to or emanate from substance use are also related to adversity and poor outcomes for parents, families and communities. However, if substance use is detected early and treated collaboratively in a multidisciplinary context, interventions are likely to have a ripple effect far beyond the individual but also facilitating the normal potential for development.[2,56–58]

REFERENCES

1 Wu P, Hoven CW, Fuller CJ. Factors associated with adolescents receiving drug treatment: findings from the National Household Survey on Drug Abuse. *Journal of Behavioral Health Services & Research.* 2003; **30**: 190–201.

2 Crome I, Chambers P, Frisher M, *et al.* 2009 *The Relationship between Dual Diagnosis: substance use and dealing with mental health issues* (SCIE Research Briefing 30). Available at: www.scie.org.uk/publications/briefings/briefing30/index.asp (accessed 23 June 2010).

3 Frisher M, Crome I, Martino O, *et al.* Epidemiology of substance use and psychiatric mental health–substance use in primary care. In: MacGregor S, editor. *Responding to Drug Misuse: research and policy priorities in health and social care.* London: Routledge; 2009.

4 Dennis ML, Scott CK, Funk R, *et al.* The duration and correlates of addiction treatment careers. *Journal of Substance Abuse Treatment.* 2005; **28**: S51–2.

5 Fuller E, editor. *Drug Use, Smoking and Drinking among Young People in England in 2007.* London: The Health and Social Care Information Centre; 2008.

6 Murphy R, Roe S. *Drug Use Declared: findings from the 2006/07 British Crime Survey – England and Wales.* London: Home Office; 2007.

7 Prime Minister's Strategy Unit. *Alcohol Harm Reduction Strategy for England.* London: Cabinet Office; 2004. Available at: www.cabinetoffice.gov.uk/media/cabinetoffice/strategy/assets/caboffce%20alcoholhar.pdf (accessed 23 June 2010).

8 Crome IB, Munafo M. Tobacco epidemiology: extent and nature of the problem. In: Ghodse H, editor. *Substance Abuse: evidence and experience in psychiatry.* London: Wiley-Blackwell; in press.

9 Action on Smoking and Health; 2009. *Essential Information on Young People and Smoking.* Available at: www.ash.org.uk/files/documents/ASH_108.pdf (accessed 23 June 2010).

10 Office for National Statistics. *Smoking Habits in Great Britain.* Cardiff: Office for National Statistics; 2009. Available at: www.statistics.gov.uk/pdfdir/nsd0309.pdf (accessed 19 July 2010).

11 DiFranza JR, Guerrera MP. Alcoholism and smoking. *Journal of Studies on Alcohol.* 1990; **51**: 130–5.

12 Wellman RJ, DiFranza JR, Savageau JA, *et al.* Short term patterns of early smoking acquisition. *Tobacco Control.* 2004; **13**: 251–7.

13 Khuder SA, Dayal HH, Mutgi AB. Age at smoking onset and its effect on smoking cessation. *Addictive Behaviors.* 1999; **24**: 673–7.

14 Karp I, O'Loughlin J, Paradis G, *et al.* Smoking trajectories of adolescent novice smokers in a longitudinal study of tobacco use. *Annals of Epidemiology.* 2005; **15**: 445–52.

15 Tyas SL, Pederson LL. Psychosocial factors related to adolescent smoking: a critical review of the literature. *Tobacco Control.* 1998; **7**: 409–20.

16 Patton GC, Carlin JB, Coffey C, et al. Depression, anxiety and smoking initiation. *American Journal of Public Health.* 1998; **90**: 1518–22.

17 Vega WA, Gil AG. Revisiting drug progression: long range effects of early tobacco use. *Addiction.* 2005; **100**: 1358–69.

18 Orlando M, Tucker JS, Ellickson PL, *et al.* Concurrent use of alcohol and cigarettes from adolescence to young adulthood: an examination of developmental trajectories and outcomes. *Substance Use and Misuse.* 2005; **40**: 1051–69.

19 Hoffman JH, Welte JW, Barnes GM. Co-occurrence of alcohol and cigarette use among adolescents. *Addictive Behaviours.* 20001; **26**: 63–78.

20 Myers MG, Kelly JF. Cigarette smoking among adolescents with alcohol and other drug use problems. *Alcohol Research and Health.* 2006; **29**: 221–7.

21 Brown RA, Lewinsohn PM, Seeley JR, *et al.* Cigarette smoking, major depression and other psychiatric disorder among adolescents. *Journal of the American Academy of Child and Adolescent Psychiatry.* 1996; **35**: 1602–10.

22 Myers MG, Brown SA. Smoking and health in substance abusing adolescents: a two year follow up. *Pediatrics.* 1994; **93**: 561–6.

23 Carra G, Johnson S. Variations in rates of comorbid substance use in psychosis between mental health settings and geographical areas in the UK. *Society of Psychiatry and Psychiatric Epidemiology.* 2009; **44**: 429–47.

24 Boys A, Farrell M, Taylor C, *et al.* Psychiatric morbidity and substance use in young people aged 13–15 years: results from the Child and Adolescent Survey of Mental Health. *British Journal of Psychiatry.* 2003; **182**: 509–17.

25 Frisher M, Crome I, Macleod J, *et al. Predictive Factors for Illicit Drug Use among Young People: a literature review* (Home Office Online Report 05/07). London: Home Office; 2007. Available at: http://rds.homeoffice.gov.uk/rds/pdfs07/rdsolr0507.pdf (accessed 23 June 2010).

26 Advisory Council on the Misuse of Drugs. *Pathways to Problems: hazardous use of tobacco, alcohol and other drugs by young people in the UK and its implications for policy.* London: Advisory Council on the Misuse of Drugs; 2006. Available at: www.homeoffice.gov.uk/publications/drugs/acmd1/pathways-to-problems/Pathwaystoproblems.pdf?view=Binary (accessed 23 June 2010).

27 Macleod J, Oakes R, Copello A, *et al.* The psychological and social sequelae of use of cannabis and other illicit drugs by young people: systematic review of longitudinal, general population studies. *Lancet.* 2004; **363**: 1579–88.

28 Beckett H, Heap J, McArdle P, *et al. Understanding Problem Drug Use among Young People Accessing Drug Services: a multivariate approach using statistical modelling techniques* (Home Office Online Report 15/04); 2004. Available at: www.homeoffice.gov.uk/rds/pdfs04/rdsolr1504.pdf (accessed 23 June 2010).

29 Raw M, McNeill A, West R. Smoking cessation guidelines for health professionals: a guide to effective smoking cessation interventions for the health care system. *Thorax.* 1998; **53**(Suppl. 5): S1–18.

30 Crome I, Bloor R, Frisher M. Editorial: self-harm and substance use in the UK – key issues for treatment and research. *Drugs: Education, Prevention and Policy.* 2008; **15**: 121–7.

31 Smith I, Crome IB. In the coroner's chair: substance use and suicide in young people – have we got the balance right? *Criminal Behaviour and Mental Health.* 2007; **17**: 197–203.

32 Myers MG, Brown SA. A controlled study of a cigarette smoking cessation intervention for adolescents in substance abuse treatment. *Psychology of Addictive Behaviours.* 2005; **19**: 230–3.

33 Cornelius JR, Maisto SA, Martin CS, *et al.* Major depression associated with earlier alcohol relapse in treated teens with AUD. *Addictive Behaviors.* 2004; **29**: 1035–8.

34 Jaycox LH, Morral AR, Juvonen J. Mental health and medical problems and service use among adolescent substance users. *Journal of the American Academy of Child and Adolescent Psychiatry.* 2003; **42**: 701–9.

35 Kelly TM, Cornelius JR, Clark DB. Psychiatric disorders and attempted suicide among adolescents with substance use disorders. *Drug and Alcohol Dependence.* 2004; **73**: 87–97.

36 Chung T, Maisto SA. Relapse to alcohol and other drug use in treated adolescents: review and reconsideration of relapse as a change point in clinical course. *Clinical Psychology Review.* 2006; **26**: 149–61.

37 Chung T, Maisto SA, Cornelius JR, *et al.* Adolescents' drug and alcohol use trajectories in the year following treatment. *Journal of Studies on Alcohol.* 2004; **65**: 105–14.

38 Chan Y, Dennis ML, Funk RR. Prevalence and mental health–substance use of major internalizing and externalizing problems among adolescents and adults presenting to substance abuse treatment. *Journal of Substance Abuse Treatment.* 2008; **34**: 14–24.

39 Shin S, Lundgren L, Chassler D. Examining drug treatment entry patterns among young injection drug users. *American Journal on Drug and Alcohol Abuse.* 2007; **33**: 217–25.

40 Dennis M, Godley SH, Diamond G, *et al.* The Cannabis Youth Treatment (CYT) Study: main findings from two randomized trials. *Journal of Substance Abuse Treatment.* 2004; **27**: 197–213.

41 Henggeler SW, Halliday-Boykins CA, Cunningham PB, *et al.* Juvenile drug court: enhancing outcomes by integrating evidence-based treatments. *Journal of Consulting and Clinical Psychology.* 2006; **74**: 42–54.

42 Molgaard V, Kumpfer KL, Spoth R. *The Iowa Strengthening Families Program for Pre- and Early Teens.* Ames, IA: Iowa State University; 1994.

43 Spoth R, Redmond C, Shin C, *et al.* Brief family intervention effects on adolescent substance initiation: school-level growth curve analyses 6 years following baseline. *Journal of Consulting and Clinical Psychology.* 2004; **72**: 535–42.

44 Waldron HB, Kern-Jones S, Turner CW, *et al.* Engaging resistant adolescents in drug abuse treatment. *Journal of Substance Abuse Treatment.* 2007; **32**: 133–42.

45 Latimer, WW, Newcomb M, Winters KC, *et al.* Adolescent substance abuse treatment outcome: the role of substance abuse problem severity, psychosocial, and treatment factors. *Journal of Consulting and Clinical Psychology.* 2000; **68**: 684–96.

46 Rowe CL, Liddle HA, Greenbaum PE, *et al.* Impact of psychiatric mental health substance use on treatment of adolescent drug users. *Journal of Substance Abuse Treatment.* 2004; **26**: 129–40.

47 White AM, Jordan JD, Schroeder KM, *et al.* Predictors of relapse during treatment and treatment completion among marijuana-dependent adolescents in an intensive outpatient substance abuse program. *Substance Abuse.* 2004; **25**: 53–9.

48 Turkington A, Mulholland CC. Impact of persistent substance use on 1 year outcome in first episode psychosis. *British Journal of Psychiatry.* 2009; **195**: 242–8.

49 Wade D, Harrigan S, Burgess PM. Substance use in first episode psychosis: 15 month prospective follow up study. *British Journal of Psychiatry.* 2006; **189**: 229–34.

50 Hides L, Dawe S, Kavanagh DJ. Psychotic symptom and cannabis relapse in recent onset psychosis. *British Journal of Psychiatry.* 2006; **189**: 137–43.

51 Green AI, Tohen MF, Hamer RM, *et al.* First episode schizophrenia-related psychosis and substance use disorders: acute response to olanzapine and haloperidol. *Schizophrenia Research.* 2004; **66**: 125–35.

52 Myers MG, Brown SA. Cigarette smoking for years following treatment for adolescent substance abuse. *Journal of Child and Adolescent Substance Abuse.* 1997; **7**: 1–15.

53 Myers MG, Macpherson L. Smoking cessation efforts among substance abusing adolescents. *Drug and Alcohol Dependence.* 2004; **73**: 209–13.

54 Knudsen HK. Adolescent only substance abuse treatment: availability and adoption of components of quality. *Journal of Substance Abuse Treatment.* 2009; **36**: 195–204.

55 Xie H, Drake R, McHugo G. Are there distinctive trajectory groups in substance misuse remission over 10 years? An application of the group based modeling. *Administration and Policy in Mental Health.* 2006; **33**: 423–32.

56 Hodges C-L, Paterson S, Taikato M, *et al. Co-morbid Mental Health and Substance Use in Scotland.* Edinburgh: Scottish Executive; 2006.

57 Advisory Council on the Misuse of Drugs. *Hidden Harm.* London: Home Office; 2003. Available at: www.drugscope.org.uk/OneStopCMS/Core/CrawlerResourceServer.aspx?resource=D5DC9EDC-E28E-4BF1-864F-75C7C456552D&mode=link&guid=9def23f124c740c886dfd52e028c16a7 (accessed 23 June 2010).

58 Advisory Council on the Misuse of Drugs. *Hidden Harm – Three Years On: realities, challenges and opportunities.* London: Advisory Council on the Misuse of Drugs; 2007.

TO LEARN MORE

- National Institute for Health and Clinical Excellence: www.nice.org.uk/
- National Institute on Drug Abuse, USA: www.nida.nih.gov/
- Substance Abuse and Mental Health Services Administration: www.samsha.gov/

CHAPTER 7

The child's perspective

Philip D James and Bobby P Smyth

INTRODUCTION

When considering mental health–substance use problems it is tempting to exclude children. To do so is a mistake. The issue of mental health–substance use can affect the child in two ways:

1 Children can experience mental health problems. Children can experience substance use problems. Therefore, it is possible for children to have the two concurrently. Even if they do not have both diagnoses in childhood, there is the question of whether the presence of one diagnosis predisposes the child to the other, consequently, developing mental health–substance use problems in the future.

2 Children can be raised by parents experiencing mental health–substance use problems that will impact on the child.

KEY POINT 7.1

A child can be defined as a young person who has not reached the age of 13.

SELF-ASSESSMENT EXERCISE 7.1

Time: 15 minutes
- Consider the causes or trigger factors for mental health–substance use in children.
- Before reading on, what do you think the figures might be? How many children are affected by experiencing mental health–substance use problems?
- Consider the impact of parental mental health–substance use problems.

CHILDREN EXPERIENCING MENTAL HEALTH OR SUBSTANCE USE PROBLEMS

The authors were unable to identify any research on the rates of mental health–substance use among children. However, there has been increasing interest in mental health–substance use problems among adolescents (*see* Book 3, Chapter 6) that may give us cause for concern. To gain an understanding of the situation we will look at the research on mental health and substance use problems among children separately. We know from international research that there is a considerable amount of mental health problems affecting children in Western society.[1] In the UK, for example, a large government study in 1999 found that among 5- to 10-year-old children 3.3% have an emotional disorder while 4.6% suffered from a form of conduct disorder.[1] One study suggests that 8.2% of children aged 5 to 10 are experiencing some form of significant mental health problem with rates of 10.4% and 5.9% found among boys and girls respectively.[1] Unfortunately, the situation does not improve with age as 11.2% of children aged between 11 and 15 experience mental health problems. The reality is many children experiencing mental health problems in childhood will go on to experience mental health problems into adolescence, and possibly adulthood. The onset at a younger age is generally regarded as being associated with a poorer prognosis.

A Scottish study examined the level of exposure to drugs among 1202 children aged 10–12, and found that almost a third had been exposed to drugs with 30.6% in situations where drugs were being used, while 14.5% had been offered drugs.[2] Cannabis (25%) and solvents (11.8%) were the most common drugs the children were exposed to and that exposure was linked with peer and family use, peer and child problem behaviours, and child alcohol use.[2] A subsequent analysis highlights the fact that the children report drugs, particularly cannabis, as being readily obtainable, and boredom as being the most common reason for using drugs along with enjoying the 'buzz' associated with the substance.[3] Moreover, they report that the main approach to avoid coming into contact with drugs was avoiding certain individuals or groups. However, this was particularly difficult to deal with when a friend started using drugs.[4] A recent World Health Organization survey reports that there is considerable variance in the rates of substance use among children worldwide.[5] For example, the percentage of children who report starting smoking by age 13 ranges from 9% in Israel to 54% in Estonia. There is a large difference between countries, with Canada and the USA both reporting rates of less than 20%, while many European countries report rates in excess of 30%, e.g. Ireland, Germany, the Netherlands and Finland. Early initiation to smoking is predictive of alcohol problems in adolescents and illicit drug problems in later life.[5] This survey demonstrates that, on average, 5% of 11-year-olds worldwide drink alcohol at least once a week and that the rates of use are higher for boys than girls (7% and 3% respectively). The rate of alcohol use tends to grow as the children move into adolescence with 11% of 13-year-olds and 26% of 15-year-olds reporting alcohol use on a weekly basis. Interestingly, these figures hide a more dramatic threefold increase in the rate of alcohol use among girls, from 3% at age 11 to 9% at age 13. By comparison, during this two-year period the rate of alcohol use among boys does not double.[5] By age 15 over 21% of girls and 31% of boys drink weekly with particularly high rates of use among some countries, such as England, Malta, Wales and Austria, and low rates in the USA, Poland, Norway and Finland. On average, 18% of 15-year-olds have used cannabis in their lifetime while a third of these have used cannabis in the past 30 days. Canada (14%) and USA (12%) top the table of regular cannabis users while

5% of Canadians and 4% of Spanish and Swiss 15-year-olds were defined as heavy users.[5] The European School Survey Project on Alcohol and other Drugs was last completed in 2007, among 15- and 16-year-olds, and found that on average across Europe 14% reported having been drunk, 7% smoking daily and 4% had tried cannabis at age 13 or younger.[6] Regarding the use of inhalants, it has been found that there is considerable variance in their use across Europe. On average, 9% of respondents had used inhalants in their lifetime with little variance overall between the genders. However, there were differences reported in individual countries.[6] Of the 9%, only one third had used them on three or more occasions and 4% had commenced use before age 14.[6] This suggests that only about 5% of students have used them regularly and that they are often used in early adolescence.

MENTAL HEALTH–SUBSTANCE USE

There are a considerable number of mental health–substance use problems among children, and these problems appear to become more common as the children become teenagers. There is much debate within the professional literature regarding the relationship between an individual's mental health and substance use problems. Does mental illness beget substance use problems or vice versa? Depression among adolescents coexists with substance use problems in up to 35% of cases, while among those with attention deficit hyperactivity disorder some studies have found no link. Other studies have reported elevated rates of substance use problems.[7,8] Conduct disorder has been reported in up to 60% of adolescents experiencing substance use problems.[8] A study of 91 teenagers aged between 13 and 18 who were receiving treatment for substance abuse found that 63.7% had a mental health problem, with depression (24%), conduct disorder (24%) and attention deficit hyperactivity disorder (11%) the most common.[9] Other estimates suggest that 50%–90% of teenagers experiencing substance use problems have a comorbid psychiatric disorder.[7] This suggests that when working with adolescents experiencing substance use problems, the presence of a psychiatric disorder is the norm and not the exception.[8] The research suggests that having a mental illness makes one more prone to developing a substance use problem.[10]

These figures are based upon research for teenagers and not children. Also, while these studies would suggest that mental health and substance use frequently coexist they do not confirm the direction of causality. Interestingly, one study found that, in general, boys tend to be diagnosed with a substance use problem, and are later diagnosed with the psychiatric disorder, while in girls the reverse is true.[11] Research would also suggest that being male and having a diagnosis of attention deficit hyperactivity disorder is associated with poorer outcome when treating the substance use problem.[9] Receiving diagnoses within a three-month period was associated with better treatment initiation and engagement compared to those who took over six months to receive their diagnoses, emphasising the need for services to actively assess and identify the presence of additional disorders.[11] A finding that underscores the importance of treating mental health–substance use effectively is that among opiate-dependent individuals, who typically have one of the poorest quality-of-life scores in society, having a concurrent mental illness is associated with a poorer quality of life.[12]

Substance use increases the likelihood of developing mental illness, and vice versa.

As in all aspects of mental healthcare the importance of exploring family history during assessment has been borne out by various research findings. Not only does the level of substance use among biological parents lead to a greater risk of developing a substance use problem but so does the level of substance use among non-biological caregivers.[10] A follow-up at 6 and 12 months on adolescents who had received treatment for substance abuse found that the children of substance-using parents tended to enter treatment with more serious problems than those of non-substance-using parents. However, they had a larger response to treatment and, at follow-up, had reduced the gap on those without substance-using parents.[13]

Young people experiencing attention deficit hyperactivity disorder are at a high risk of developing a substance use problem in life.[14,15] The link between attention deficit hyperactivity disorder and substance use problems appears to be particularly strong if the individual also has conduct disorder, and not treating the attention deficit hyperactivity disorder tends to lead to poorer outcomes.[15] It is established through rigorous research that the best outcomes in attention deficit hyperactivity disorder involves the use of medication.[16] However, there has been concern about treating individuals experiencing attention deficit hyperactivity disorder who are using substances with medications, because psycho-stimulants, the main medications used in the treatment of attention deficit hyperactivity disorder, have themselves the potential for misuse. A literature review found that the use of medications in the treatment of attention deficit hyperactivity disorder does not increase the risk of substance misuse.[15] Another study completed a meta-analysis that found children with attention deficit hyperactivity disorder treated with psycho-stimulants are less likely to develop substance use problems than those who are not, suggesting that failure to treat attention deficit hyperactivity disorder is the problem.[17] A trial of a psycho-stimulant (pemoline) for adolescents with attention deficit hyperactivity disorder and substance use problems found that while it did have a positive impact on attention deficit hyperactivity disorder symptoms it did not improve the substance use problem or conduct disorder symptoms.[18] Cases of adults with attention deficit hyperactivity disorder–substance use problems who were successfully treated using psycho-stimulants are described within the literature.[14] However, some confusing advice is evident. Randomised controlled trials have shown that the use of psycho-stimulants can work for those experiencing attention deficit hyperactivity disorder and substance use problems but appear to recommend withholding stimulants until after a period of abstinence.[15] As stimulants work for those with co-occurring substance use problems[15,17,18] it would appear to make more sense to provide appropriate medication for the attention deficit hyperactivity disorder. This may make the individual more amenable to the normal psychological treatments used in substance use problems, such as motivational interviewing (see Book 4, Chapter 7). If misuse of the prescribed medication is a concern, the prescriber should be vigilant of lost prescriptions and parents or guardians can take responsibility for dispensing the medication as prescribed.[15]

There will be some children who are using drugs and naturally some of these may have psychiatric disorders. It is possible that children will not present with a mental health–substance use problem until adolescence. However, a psychiatric diagnosis in childhood appears to increase the risk of developing a substance use problem. Therefore, children with psychiatric disorders are at high risk of developing mental health–substance use problems. Moreover, research indicates that those who are treated for a substance use problem often have undiagnosed mental illness. Professionals working with children with mental health problems should routinely assess for the presence of a substance use problem(s), and vice versa, as the identification of the two (or more) problems close together appears to be a positive indicator of outcome.[11] Once a child is identified as experiencing mental health–substance use problems the question then turns to treatment.

There appears to be no research on how to treat children experiencing mental health–substance use problems. In adolescents having a psychiatric disorder is associated with poorer engagement and outcome in treatment of a substance use problem and so the presence of mental health–substance use problems needs to be identified quickly and targeted for treatment.[9,11] Two recent reviews have examined the issue of treating mental health–substance use problems, though not specifically with young people.[19,20] One found that treatments that are known to work in mental illness (e.g. antidepressants) and substance use (e.g. motivational interviewing) tend to work in those experiencing mental health–substance use problems.[19] Interestingly, they found that there was little evidence supporting integrated treatments. Motivational interviewing was found to have the most evidence to support its efficacy in reducing substance use in the short term, and when combined with cognitive behavioural therapy it had a positive effect on mental state.[20] However, cognitive behavioural therapy alone was not effective and contingency management and longer-term residential programmes have some promising evidence supporting their use but the evidence is still rather weak and further robust research is required.[20]

KEY POINT 7.3

When mental health and substance use problems coexist they appear to impact on each other. Early intervention and active planning addressing both is paramount.

CHILDREN OF PARENTS EXPERIENCING MENTAL HEALTH–SUBSTANCE USE PROBLEMS

From a child's perspective the quality of the parenting they receive is of paramount importance as it exerts considerable influence on an individual's functioning later in life.[21–24] It is for this reason that we must look at the issue of being raised by a parent experiencing mental health–substance use problems. The authors were unable to identify any research on the specific effect of mental health–substance use on an individual's ability to parent, or on outcomes for their children. However, there is some research examining the effect of parental mental health and substance use problems on children.

CHILDREN OF SUBSTANCE-USING PARENTS

There is generally a degree of concern for the welfare of children in society and, therefore, considerable attention has been paid to the children of people who use substances. The issue was firmly in the spotlight in the UK following the high-profile trial of a heroin-dependent man for the murder of his girlfriend's (also heroin-dependent) son. Headlines such as '*Drug abuse and parenting don't mix*'[25] and '*Drug addicts' children should be adopted*'[26] appeared in national papers. There are a number of research papers examining the effects of having a parent experiencing substance use problems. A research overview suggested that the children of 'alcoholics' have been shown to have poorer outcomes than the general population in terms of social, educational and substance use.[27] However, little research had been undertaken on the children of opiate, cocaine and poly-drug users.[27] A more recent review suggests that the role of maternal substance use problems needs to be examined further as there has been a focus on paternal use over the preceding years.[28] One study suggests that there is a need to research 'alcoholic and drug abusing parents' separately as illegal drugs are generally associated with more criminal problems, social isolation, stigma and secrecy, which are likely to have a severe effect on the children.[28] This matter is further complicated by the reality that a large number of people who misuse drugs also misuse alcohol. They conclude that there is strong evidence that children living within this environment are prone to a variety of risks and recommend that more programmes are needed that help address these risks.[28]

A number of studies examine the effects of poly-drug-using parents on their children.[13,29-31] A comparison of 20 children of drug-'abusing' parents and 20 controls found that a negative and depressive attributional style was more common among the offspring of parents experiencing substance use problems.[29] One study examined the effects of parental substance use problems on children (mean age 15.9) and found children were at an elevated risk of developing a substance use problem as an adolescent.[30] However, while exposure to parental substance use problems in childhood conferred a two-fold increase in risk of developing a substance use problem, exposure during adolescence carried a three-fold increase in risk, suggesting that adolescents who are exposed to parental substance use problems are at particular risk.[30] This mirrors previous findings that the effects of a father's substance use problems had a greater risk for sons the later in childhood they were exposed to it.[32] Another study examined 255 college students (49% female), and found that their current levels of psychological distress was more closely related to parental emotional abuse as a child than specific reports of either childhood sexual abuse or parental substance use problems.[31] However, one should be cautious in generalising these findings widely as college students may not be representative of the majority of childhood sexual abuse victims or children of people who use substances. Another study found that adolescent children of people who use substances, who themselves received treatment for substance use problems, tended to enter with more severe problems.[13] However, this did not negatively affect their outcome.[13] They tended to show 'bigger gains' from treatment and, therefore, closed the gap on the children of non-substance-using parents.

Interviews with 70 opiate-using parents (36 women, of 188 children) who were receiving methadone maintenance found that:

- 64% of mothers admitted to using psychoactive drugs during their pregnancy
- 80% of parents had been arrested during their child's life
- 7% of parents reported their child had experienced childhood sexual abuse
- 9% had had charges of neglect or physical abuse directed towards them.[33]

These parents also reported that their children were displaying numerous problems, including:
- truancy (19%)
- suspension from school (30%)
- contact with the law (12%)
- involved with drugs or alcohol (17%)
- discipline problems (29%).

Another study followed up 67 children of opiate users (aged 3–14) who were living with their opiate-addicted parent at least half the time and found that:
- 70% had at least one change in who was completing either the mother or father role
- a quarter did not have a stable parent for the duration of the study[34]
- parent figure transitions and parental criminality were each associated with delinquent behaviour in the children.[34]

FATHERS EXPERIENCING SUBSTANCE USE PROBLEMS

There has been a considerable amount of attention paid towards sons of substance-using fathers. One study found that the sons (age 10 to 12 years) of poly-substance-using fathers were found to:
- exhibit more internalising (e.g. sadness and worry) behaviours
- exhibit more externalising (e.g. aggression) behaviours
- have lower IQ and poorer school achievement, when scores were controlled for socioeconomic status.[35]

School achievement and IQ scores were more strongly associated with paternal substance use problems while internalising and externalising scores were more strongly associated with having two substance-using parents.[35] A number of subsequent studies by the same authors examined the salivary cortisol responses of sons of substance abusers. The hypothalamic-pituitary-adrenal cortical axis is typically activated during acute stress, but individuals who have been repeatedly exposed to acute stresses exhibit an attenuated response.[36] Sons of poly-substance-using fathers have a reduced cortisol response when exposed to stress compared to control groups.[37] The later in the son's life the father's substance use problems commenced the greater the effect on the cortisol response, with the greatest effect in those whose father's substance use problems commenced in the previous two years.[36] Those sons whose fathers developed their substance use problems prior to age three displayed the same cortisol levels as those whose fathers never experienced a substance use problem.[36] When a father's substance use problem ceases before the son's sixth birthday they are at no more at risk of internalising or externalising psychopathology than controls.[32] However, when the substance use extends beyond the sixth birthday the sons become at increased risk of displaying such psychopathology.[32] On a positive note, research has shown that treating a father's 'alcoholism' leads to significant reduction in child problems.[38]

Preadolescent tobacco use and early adolescent regular alcohol use were associated with the presence of paternal substance use problems and conduct disorder.[39] One study examined 120 families with both parents living with an 8–12-year-old child divided evenly between three subgroups:

1   Drug-abusing fathers
2   Alcohol-abusing fathers
3   Non-substance-abusing fathers.[40]

They found that children from drug-abusing families reported the most internalising and externalising symptoms, while those from alcohol-abusing families displayed more symptoms than those from non-addicted families.[40] According to parents' reports the children in the drug-using families were also exposed to more physical violence and marital conflict. Fathers from these families were more likely to report 'dysfunctional parenting practices' and to engage in less supervision of their children, while mothers' parenting practices were not significantly different across the three family types.[40] All these studies suggest that children raised in families where the father is using substances are more likely to suffer from psychiatric symptoms and inappropriate substance use themselves. Moreover, having a father who is using cocaine or opiates appears to be a greater risk factor than alcohol-related problems. Higher levels of psychosocial maladjustment are associated with parents' younger age, lower incomes, emotional distress and frequency of fathers' substance use.[41] However, aggression by fathers towards mothers was the variable that exerted the most negative influence on the children's adjustment.[41]

KEY POINT 7.4

A parent's substance use appears to elevate the risk of poorer psychosocial outcomes for the child.

PARENTS EXPERIENCING MENTAL HEALTH–SUBSTANCE USE PROBLEMS

There appears to be no research that specifically looks at the effects of a parent experiencing mental health–substance use problems. However, some of the studies examining parents with either substance use or mental health problems make reference to the other. In a sample of 70 opiate-using mothers and fathers in the USA, it was found that 34% reported having treatment for an emotional disorder, with 14% receiving inpatient psychiatric treatment.[33] One study examined the personality characteristics of young adult children of substance users and found:

➤   a considerable variance in the rates of abuse/neglect among children whose parents had no psychological difficulties (20%)
➤   other psychological problems, mainly depression and anxiety disorders (39%)

➤ substance-using parents (53%)
➤ mental health–substance use problems (65%).[42]

Depression and neuroticism were more related to the level of abuse and neglect experienced by the individual rather than their parents' diagnosis,[42] suggesting that the children of parents experiencing a mental health–substance use problem are more at risk than children of either substance misusers or those with emotional problems. Another study examining the characteristics of mothers who were in contact with both mental health services and child protection services found that poly-substance use (39.3%) and mental health–substance use problems (19.7%) were the most common diagnosis.[43]

LIMITATIONS

When considering the literature related to the children of substance-using parents one should be mindful of an important critique of this area. While many articles examine the effects of parental substance use problems on their children, it is probably a mistake to assume that the effect of parental substance use will be the same regardless of the substance being used. Cocaine and opiate users for example are more likely to:

➤ live in poverty
➤ be involved in criminal activities
➤ have drug use problems associated with more complicated health problems such as HIV.[28,44]

As alcohol problems among cocaine and opiate users are so common it would be unrepresentative to have a sample comprised solely of drug-using fathers who were not also experiencing alcohol-related problems.[40]

CHILDREN LIVING ALONGSIDE SUBSTANCE-USING PARENTS

Much of the harm experienced by children of substance-using parents comes not from the substance use per se, but from the high risk of suffering neglect.[45] Children raised in families with parents experiencing mental health–substance use problems are at increased risk of abuse and neglect,[42,43] and it is this neglect, regardless of its links to substance use or mental illness, that places the child at risk of developing a variety of psychosocial problems. Numerous articles summarise various community and residential programmes aimed at providing support and intervention to drug-using parents, particularly mothers and their children.[46,47] However, trying to work with the individual who uses drugs regarding their parenting provides numerous challenges, including promoting honesty and openness, while also dealing appropriately with abuse and neglect.[46] While many of these programmes appear interesting, there is no strong evidence to support their effectiveness, and given the large number of children living with parents who use substances there is a need for effective and efficient interventions to be identified.[47] Barnard and McKeganey provide an overview of a number of these interventions and programmes including:

➤ Focus on Families – provides a combination of small group training to parents and home care.

➤ The Nurturing Programme – delivered training for 2.5 hours per week for 23 weeks to pregnant women or mothers as part of a residential programme.
➤ Home visiting – trained community health nurses provide support and advocacy to drug-using women from pregnancy until the child is 18 months. Staff provided two one-hour visits per week.
➤ The Seattle Birth to Three programme – a home visiting programme provided by trained paraprofessionals who visited up to twice weekly as needed until the child was three years old.

One example of a promising approach is teaching parenting skills to parents attending methadone clinics, which has been shown to improve parenting skills and knowledge.[48] However, a dilemma will always remain because while some drug-using parents might improve, there will always be some whose substance use will continue to place their children at considerable risk. There is a need to develop measures to ensure that children who live with substance-using parents are protected.[49] These measures can include:
➤ improving the quality of parenting
➤ education and training of professionals working with those experiencing mental health–substance use problems.

However, a balance may need to be struck here as some people may be dissuaded from accessing treatment if they believed that their parenting skills are likely to come under scrutiny when they seek treatment for substance use problems.

SELF-ASSESSMENT EXERCISE 7.2

Time: 10 minutes
How, as a professional, might you manage to balance the needs of the family against the possibility of alienating them?

CHILDREN LIVING ALONGSIDE PARENTS EXPERIENCING MENTAL HEALTH PROBLEMS

For decades we have known that children of parents with mental illness are at increased risk of a range of psychosocial outcomes[50] including increased rates of death by unnatural causes.[51] A recent review of the offspring of individuals experiencing bipolar affective disorder highlighted the high levels of mental health problems among their children, with one study reporting that 40% of parents experiencing bipolar affective disorders have at least one child who received some type of mental health service.[52] Another study found that over half of people attending an adult mental health service had children, but only 32% of those with a diagnosis of schizophrenia had children compared to 68% and 60% of those diagnosed with depression and bipolar affective disorder respectively.[53] A study on the outcomes of adult children of mothers with serious mental illness found that in about one-third of cases the children had not completed secondary-level education, and over half had a serious psychological, legal or substance use problem with a maternal diagnosis of bipolar affective disorder particularly associated with problems.[54] Children of parents who are hospitalised for psychiatric treatment have been shown to experience depression and anxiety scores within the normal range.[55] This gives credence to the assertion that it is not the acute psychiatric episode that causes childhood difficulties but rather the chronic neglect and poor parenting that may go with having a parent with a mental health problem.[53]

SELF-ASSESSMENT EXERCISE 7.3

Time: 15 minutes

Taking the concept of resilience, applied to your own character, consider what makes you resilient when dealing with children and families in perpetual distress.

From the research, the concept of resilience has emerged whereby numerous factors in the child, the parent, and their social network help to protect the child from developing difficulties, including mental illness.[50,56] These protective factors include temperament, social and intellectual abilities, parenting skills and the presence of a positive relationship with at least one parent and external adult role models. The identification of these factors suggests that interventions aimed at boosting a child's resilience in the face of their parents' mental illness could be effective. A recent study showed how a 10-session cognitive behavioural therapy intervention for at-risk adolescents with alcohol-dependent parents was successful in increasing their resilience.[57] Therefore, adult mental health services should enquire about the children of individuals attending their service, aiming to identify those who may benefit from support.[50,52-54] However, assuming the children of those with mental illnesses who are most at risk are identified, what can be done to help them? Two broad methods have been suggested:

1 Programmes should be developed which develop the child and parents' ability to cope as well as pulling in other resources within the extended family.[58]
2 Work needs to be done to bring together the various professionals and services who are working with the family, such as general practitioners, mental health, social services, educational, etc., to allow for a more coordinated and family-friendly service.[58]

However, while a recent study demonstrated promising results in developing resilience in children of alcohol-dependent parents,[57] another with children of those with a mental illness was not as successful.[59] A number of projects aimed at developing the quality of parenting among those with substance use problems have been developed over a number of years, and many are showing considerable potential. These include:

➤ Home Intervention[60]
➤ Parents Under Pressure programme[61]
➤ Partners in Parenting[62]
➤ The Mothers and Toddlers Programme.[63]

> **KEY POINT 7.5**

The child's outcome will improve by
- improving the child's quality of life
- increasing parenting skills
- decreasing parental mental health–substance use symptoms
- increasing the child's resilience.

CONCLUSIONS

SELF-ASSESSMENT EXERCISE 7.4

Time: 30 minutes
- After reviewing the literature, what conclusions can be made?
- What proposals in your service could be made?
- How could change in your service be implemented?
- What policy guidelines would be helpful in bringing about change in your service?

Based upon the literature, the following conclusions may be drawn.
- ➤ Large numbers of children have mental health problems (particularly conduct disorder and attention deficit hyperactivity disorder) and the rates of mental illness increase as they move into adolescence.
- ➤ Many children commence using substances (usually cigarettes) before they are adolescents. This early substance use is associated with more severe substance use problems later in life.
- ➤ Adolescents experiencing mental health–substance use problems tend to be associated with poorer outcomes for both problems, particularly when one or other is not identified and treated.
- ➤ Services working with children need to be mindful that mental health–substance use problems in children are treatable.
- ➤ Children living with parents or caregivers with a mental illness or substance use problem tend to be at risk of poor psychosocial adjustment.
- ➤ The longer into the child's life the parents substance misuse persists, and the more chronic neglect they experience, the more this is associated with poor outcomes.
- ➤ Programmes to improve parenting and to increase the child's resilience are showing some positive results.

REFERENCES

1 Meltzer H, Gatward R, Goodman R, *et al. The Mental Health of Children and Adolescents in Great Britain.* London: The Stationary Office; 2000.
2 McIntosh J, Gannon M, McKeganey, N, *et al.* Exposure to drugs among pre-teenage school-children. *Addiction.* 2003; **98**: 1615–23.

3 McIntosh J, MacDonald F, McKeganey N. Pre-teenage children's experiences of drug use. *International Journal of Drug Policy.* 2005; **16**: 37–45.

4 McIntosh J, MacDonald F, McKeganey, N. Pre-teenage children's strategies for avoiding situations in which they might be exposed to drugs. *Drugs: Education, Prevention and Policy.* 2005; **12**: 5–17.

5 World Health Organization. *Inequalities in Young People's Health: health behaviours of school children international report.* Edinburgh: Child and Adolescent Health Research Unit; 2008.

6 Hibell B, Guttormson U, Ahlstrom S, *et al. The 2007 ESPAD Report: Substance Use Among Students in 35 European Countries.* Stockholm: Swedish Council for Information on Alcohol and other Drugs; 2009.

7 Solhkhah R. The intoxicated child. *Child Adolescent Psychiatric Clinics of North America.* 2003; **12**: 693–722.

8 Deas D. Adolescent substance abuse and psychiatric comorbidities. *Journal of Clinical Psychiatry.* 2006; **67**(Suppl. 7): S18–23.

9 Wise BK, Cuffe SP, Fischer T. Dual diagnosis and successful participation of adolescents in substance abuse treatment. *Journal of Substance Abuse Treatment.* 2001; **21**: 161–5.

10 Comotis KA, Tisdall WA, Holdcraft LC, *et al.* Dual diagnosis: impact of family history. *American Journal of Addiction.* 2005; **14**: 291–9.

11 Chi FW, Sterling S, Weisner C. Adolescents with co-occurring substance use and mental conditions in a private managed care health plan: prevalence, patient characteristics and treatment initiation and engagement. *American Journal of Addiction.* 2006; **15**: 67–79.

12 Bizzarri J, Rucci P, Vallotta A, *et al.* Dual diagnosis and quality of life in patients in treatment for opiate dependence. *Substance Use and Misuse.* 2005; **40**: 1765–76.

13 Leichtling G, Gabrial RM, Lewis CK, *et al.* Adolescents in treatment: effects of parental substance abuse on treatment entry characteristics and outcomes. *Journal of Social Work Practice in the Addictions.* 2006; **6**: 155–74.

14 Schubiner H, Tzelpis A, Isaacson H, *et al.* The dual diagnosis of attention-deficit/hyperactivity disorder and substance abuse: care reports and literature review. *Journal of Clinical Psychiatry.* 1995; **56**: 146–50.

15 Upadhyaya HP. Substance use disorders in children and adolescents with attention-deficit/hyperactivity disorder: implications for treatment and the role of the primary care physician. *Journal of Clinical Psychiatry, Primary Care Companion.* 2008; **10**: 211–21.

16 Murray DW, Arnold LE, Swanson J, *et al.* A clinical review of outcomes of the multimodal treatment study of children with attention-deficit/hyperactivity disorder (MTA). *Current Psychiatry Reports.* 2008; **10**: 424–31.

17 Wilens TE, Faraone SV, Biederman J, *et al.* Does stimulant therapy of attention-deficit/hyperactivity disorder beget later substance abuse? A meta-analytic review of the literature. *Pediatrics.* 2003; **111**: 179–85.

18 Riggs PD, Hall SK, Mikulich-Gilbertson SK, *et al.* A randomized controlled trial of pemoline for attention-deficit-hyperactivity disorder in substance-abusing adolescents. *Journal of the American Academy of Child and Adolescent Psychiatry.* 2004; **43**: 420–9.

19 Tiet QQ, Mausbach B. Treatments for patients with dual diagnosis: a review. *Alcoholism: Clinical and Experimental Research.* 2007; **31**: 513–36.

20 Cleary M, Hunt GE, Matheson S, *et al.* Psychosocial treatments for people with co-occurring severe mental illness and substance misuse: systematic review. *Journal of Advanced Nursing.* 2009; **65**: 238–58.

21 Collins WA, Maccoby EE, Steinberg L, *et al.* Contemporary research on parenting: the case for nature and nurture. *American Journal of Psychology.* 2000; **55**: 218–32.

22 Johnson GJ, Cohen P, Gould MS, *et al*. Childhood adversities, interpersonal difficulties, and risk for suicide attempts during late adolescence and early adulthood. *Archives of General Psychiatry*. 2002; **59**: 741–9.

23 Feinberg ME, Button TMM, Neiderhiser JM, *et al*. Parenting and adolescent antisocial behaviour and depression. *Archives of General Psychiatry*. 2007; **64**: 457–65.

24 Tildesley EA, Andrews JA. The development of children's intentions to use alcohol: direct and indirect effects of parent alcohol use and parenting behaviours. *Psychology of Addictive Behaviors*. 2008; **22**: 326–39.

25 Barnard M. Drug abuse and parents don't mix. *The Sunday Times*. 8 March 2009. London. Available at: www.timesonline.co.uk/tol/news/uk/health/article5863852.ece (accessed 24 June 2010).

26 Reid M. Drug addicts' 'children should be adopted'. *The Times*. 8 March 2009. London. Available at: www.timesonline.co.uk/tol/news/uk/scotland/article5871104.ece (accessed 24 June 2010).

27 Johnson JL, Leff M. Children of substance abusers: overview of research findings. *Paediatrics*. 1999; **103**: 1085–99.

28 Schroeder V, Kelley ML, Fals-Stewart W. Effects of parental substance abuse on youth in their homes. *The Prevention Researcher*. 2006; **13**: 10–13.

29 Perez-Bouchard L, Johnson JL, Ahrens A. Attributional style in children of substance abusers. *American Journal of Drug and Alcohol Abuse*. 1993; **19**: 475–89.

30 Biederman J, Faraone SV, Monuteaux MC, *et al*. Patterns of alcohol and drug use in adolescents can be predicted by parental substance use disorders. *Pediatrics*. 2000; **106**: 792–7.

31 Melchert TP. Clarifying the effects of parental substance abuse, child sexual abuse, and parental caregiving on adult adjustment. *Professional Psychology: Research and Practice*. 2000; **31**: 64–9.

32 Moss HB, Clark DB, Kirisci L. Timing of paternal substance use disorder cessation and effects on problem behaviours in sons. *American Journal of Addiction*. 1997; **6**: 30–7.

33 Kolar AF, Brown BS, Haertzen CA, *et al*. Children of substance abusers: the life experiences of children of opiate addicts in methadone maintenance. *American Journal of Drug and Alcohol Abuse*. 1994; **20**: 159–71.

34 Keller TE, Catalano RF, Haggerty KP, *et al*. Parent figure transitions and delinquency and drug use among early adolescent children of substance abusers. *American Journal of Drug and Alcohol Abuse*. 2002; **28**: 399–427.

35 Moss HB, Vanyukov M, Majumder PP, *et al*. Prepubertal sons of substance abusers: influences of parental and familial substance abuse on behavioral disposition, IQ, and school achievement. *Addictive Behaviors*. 1995; **20**: 345–58.

36 Moss HB, Vanyukov M, Yao JK, *et al*. Salivary cortisol responses in prepubertal boys: the effects of parental substance abuse and association with drug use behaviour during adolescents. *Biological Psychiatry*. 1999; **45**: 1293–9.

37 Moss HB, Vanyukov MM, Martin CS. Salivary cortisol responses and the risk for substance abuse in prepubertal boys. *Biological Psychiatry*. 1995; **38**: 547–55.

38 Andreas JB, O'Farrell T, Fals-Stewart W. Does individual treatment for alcoholic fathers benefit their children? A longitudinal assessment. *Journal of Consulting and Clinical Psychol*. 2006; **74**: 191–8.

39 Clarke DB, Kirisci L, Moss HB. Early adolescent gateway drug use in sons of fathers with substance abuse disorders. *Addictive Behaviors*. 1998: **23**: 561–6.

40 Fals-Stewart W, Kelley ML, Fincham FD, *et al*. Emotional and behavioural problems of children living with drug-abusing fathers: comparisons with children living with

alcohol-abusing and non-substance-abusing fathers. *Journal of Family Psychology.* 2004; **18**: 319–30.

41 Fals-Stewart W, Kelley ML, Cooke CG., *et al.* Predictors of the psychosocial adjustment of children living in households of parents in which fathers abuse drugs: the effects of postnatal parental exposure. *Addictive Behaviors.* 2003; **28**: 1013–31.

42 Henderson MC, Albright JS, Kalichman SC, *et al.* Personality characteristics of young adult offspring of substance abusers: a study highlighting methodological issues. *Journal of Personality Assessment.* 1994; **63**: 117–34.

43 Lewin L, Abdrbo A. Mothers with self-reported Axis I diagnoses and child protection. *Archives of Psychiatric Nursing.* 2009; **23**: 200–9.

44 Hogan DM. Annotation: the psychological development and welfare of children of opiate and cocaine users: review and research needs. *Journal of Child Psychology and Psychiatry.* 1998; **39**: 609–20.

45 Dunn MG, Tarter RE, Mezzich AC, *et al.* Origins and consequences of child neglect in substance abuse families. *Clinical Psychology Review.* 2002; **22**: 1063–90.

46 Banwell C, Denton B, Bammer G. Programmes for the children of illicit drug-using parents: issues and dilemmas. *Drug and Alcohol Review.* 2002; **21**: 381–6.

47 Barnard M, McKeganey N. The impact of parental problem drug use on children: what is the problem and what can be done to help? *Addiction.* 2004; **99**: 552–9.

48 Gainey RR, Haggerty KP, Fleming CB, *et al.* Teaching parenting skills in a methadone maintenance setting. *Journal of Social Work Research and Evaluation.* 2007; **31**: 185–90.

49 Advisory Council on the Misuse of Drugs. *Hidden Harm: responding to the needs of children of problem drug users.* Edinburgh: Advisory Council on the Misuse of Drugs; 2002. Available at: www.drugmisuse.isdscotland.org/publications/local/hharm_full.pdf (accessed 24 June 2010).

50 Delvin JM, O'Brien LM. Children of parents with mental illness. I: An overview from a nursing perspective. *Australian and New Zealand Journal of Mental Health Nursing.* 1999; **8**: 19–29.

51 Chen YH, Chiou HY, Tang, CH, *et al.* Risk of death by unnatural causes during early childhood in offspring of parents with mental illness. *American Journal of Psychiatry.* 2010; **167**: 198–205.

52 Hodgins S, Faucher B, Zarac A, *et al.* Children of parents with bipolar disorder. A population at high risk for major affective disorder. *Child and Adolescent Psychiatry Clinics of North America.* 2002; **11**: 533–53.

53 Ahern K. At-risk children: a demographic analysis of the children of clients attending mental health community clinics. *International Journal of Mental Health Nursing.* 2002; **12**: 223–8.

54 Mowbray CT, Bybee D, Oyserman D, *et al.* Psychosocial outcomes for adult children of parents with severe mental illnesses: demographic and clinical history predictors. *Health and Social Work.* 2006; **31**: 99–108.

55 Sivec HJ, Masterson P, Katz JG, *et al.* The response of children to the psychiatric hospitalisation of a family member. *Australian e-Journal for the Advancement of Mental Health.* 2008; **7**. Available at: http://amh.e-contentmanagement.com/archives/vol/7/issue/2/article/3276/the-response-of-children-to-the-psychiatric (accessed 19 July 2010).

56 Atkinson PA, Martin CR Rankin J. Resilience revisited. *Journal of Psychiatry and Mental Health Nursing.* 2009; **16**: 137–45.

57 Hyun MS, Nam KA, Kim MA. Randomised controlled trial of a cognitive-behavioural therapy for at-risk Korean male adolescents. *Archives of Psychiatric Nursing.* 2010; **24**: 202–11.

58 Handley C, Farrell GA, Josephs A, *et al.* The Tasmanian children's project: the needs of children with a parent/carer with a mental illness. *Australian and New Zealand Journal of Mental Health Nursing.* 2001; **10**: 221–8.

59 Frazer E, Pakenham KI. Evaluation of a resilience-based intervention for children of parents with mental illness. *Australia and New Zealand Journal of Psychiatry.* 2008; **42**: 1041–50.

60 Schuler ME, Nair P, Black MM. Ongoing maternal drug use, parenting attitudes and a home intervention: effects on mother-child interaction at 18 months. *Developmental and Behavioural Pediatrics.* 2002; **23**: 87–94.

61 Dawe S, Harnett PH, Rendalls V, *et al.* Improving family functioning and child outcome in methadone maintained families: the Parents Under Pressure programme. *Drug and Alcohol Review.* 2003; **22**: 299–307.

62 Knight DK, Bartholomew NG, Simpson DD. An exploratory study of 'partners in parenting' within two substance abuse treatment programmes for women. *Psychological Services.* 2007; **4**: 262–76.

63 Suchman N, DeCoste C, Castiglioni N, *et al.* The Mothers and Toddlers Programme: preliminary findings from an attachment-based parenting intervention for substance-abusing mothers. *Psychoanalytic Psychology.* 2008; **25**: 499–517.

TO LEARN MORE

- **40 Developmental Assets**: The Search Institute is involved in developing the 40 developmental assets which are 40 common-sense, positive experiences and qualities that promote health development and reduce emotional and behavioural difficulties in children. The assets can therefore be used to inform education and preventative work with at-risk children and their parents: www.search-institute.org
- **Partners in Parenting**: An eight-session programme aimed at improving the parenting skills of parents in substance abuse treatment. The manual and other resources are available here for free download: www.ibr.tcu.edu/pubs/trtmanual/parenting.html
- **The Parents Under Pressure Programme**: The PUP programme aims to improve family functioning and child outcomes by addressing risk factors within the family and the wider social system in substance abusing families. Primarily it focuses on decreasing parental psychopathology and then to increase the quality of parenting practices. This website provides a wealth of information on this approach: www.pupprogram.net.au/

CHAPTER 8

The additive effect of mental health–substance use on cognitive impairment

Victoria CL Manning and Shai L van der Karre Betteridge

INTRODUCTION

People experiencing mental health–substance use problems can be difficult to treat.[1] The term 'revolving-door patients'[2] recognises their increased demand on services, relative to people with a single diagnosis of mental health or substance use disorder. Despite this, they tend to achieve poorer outcomes, often attributed to a lack of motivation, poor engagement in treatment and high attrition rates.[3] Level of cognitive functioning may play a mediating role in motivation to change and abstain from substance use.[4] Substance use disorders and severe mental illnesses can cause impairments in cognitive, interpersonal, affective and biological functioning.[5] Where the two co-occur, the interaction may exacerbate the nature and severity of these impairments. This chapter aims to describe the types of cognitive impairment common among individuals experiencing mental health–substance use problems, how they are identified, and how the delivery of treatment can be modified to enhance treatment outcomes.

WHAT IS COGNITIVE FUNCTIONING?

Cognition concerns the way information is collected, assimilated, organised, stored and used. 'Cognitive functioning' is an umbrella term used to refer to all activities associated with thinking and reasoning, including constructs, such as language, intelligence and memory.[6] While there is no universally recognised model of cognitive functioning, it is widely accepted that it can be subdivided into six functional domains:
1 General intellectual functioning
2 Language skills
3 Visuospatial skills
4 Attention and concentration
5 Memory and learning
6 Executive functioning.

1 General intellectual functioning

An individual's general level of intellectual functioning is perceived to be a global estimate of someone's cognitive functions.

2 Language skills

➤ Expressive language skills – ability to name objects, and the speed and ease of verbal production.

➤ Receptive language – the person's ability to comprehend auditory information.

3 Visuospatial skills

These cover a wide range of visual and perceptual abilities such as judging depth, distance and the spatial orientation of objects. These skills are used in most activities of daily living, e.g. dressing, assembling furniture, walking, driving and any other activity that involves interacting with the environment.

4 Attention and concentration

This refers to the ability to focus on visual or auditory stimuli (attention) and remain focused for a period of time (concentration).

5 Memory and learning

Memory is principally classified into retrograde memory (autobiographical information), and anterograde memory (the capacity to process and the storage of new information). The latter has the greatest impact on rehabilitative potential. It is widely accepted that memory is not one system, and terminology such as 'short-term' and 'long-term' memory are well known to the layperson. Neuropsychologists quantify long-term memory by measuring information recalled after a delay of 15–20 minutes. This model of assessment is based on information-processing models of memory,[7] which proposed that there are three mechanisms involved in the process of forming memories:

1 **Encoding**: the processes by which information is registered or translated into a mental representation based on acoustic code (how it sounds), visual code (how it looks), or semantic code (what it means). Information recalled immediately after it is presented forms a measure of how much information a person has encoded.

2 **Storage**: the maintenance of information over time. Information recalled after 15–20 minutes is thought to be in long-term memory store and therefore should be accessible days later.

3 **Retrieval**: accessing information from memory stores. This is measured by showing a person previously presented information along with distracter items, to see what is recognised or by providing cues or prompts.

Short-term memory refers to the ability to recall information immediately after presentation (e.g. a string of letters), and therefore is often viewed more as a function of attention rather than memory per se. In everyday life we use this skill as part of working memory, which refers to the ability to hold information in mind and manipulate it in order to perform a specific task (e.g. mental arithmetic, dialling a phone number, or following a set of directions). The process of mentally manipulating information when using working memory is referred to as mental flexibility, and is viewed as an aspect of executive functioning.

6 Executive functioning

This refers to higher order functions that control and regulate behaviour. They are often referred to as 'frontal functions' because they are sub-served (though not exclusively) by the frontal and prefrontal regions of the brain. Executive functions are necessary for goal-directed behaviour and include the ability to:

- formulate concepts
- think abstractly
- make decisions and to be able to weigh information
- organise, prioritise and plan
- initiate and inhibit actions
- reflect, self-monitor progress, and anticipate outcomes (especially when facing novel tasks)
- adapt behaviour to changing situations
- juggle multiple pieces of information in one's mind (mental flexibility).

Executive functions are dissociable and thus can be differentially impaired.

WHAT IS COGNITIVE IMPAIRMENT?

Cognitive impairment can be caused by:

- psychiatric illness
- substance misuse
- learning disabilities
- stress
- poor nutrition
- medication
- sleep deprivation
- genetic factors
- brain injury
- and a whole range of medical disorders.[8]

It is usually indicated by performance on neuropsychological tests falling more than one-standard deviation below that of a normal (healthy) population. However, in order to establish the extent of cognitive impairment, it is necessary to estimate the individual's level of functioning (pre-morbid IQ) prior to any decline.

EVIDENCE FOR COGNITIVE IMPAIRMENT IN PSYCHIATRIC AND SUBSTANCE USE DISORDERS

Substance use disorders

Cognitive impairment (in particular impaired decision-making, inhibition and cognitive flexibility) is thought to play a role in the development, maintenance and relapse of addictive behaviours.[9] Common behavioural dysfunction among people experiencing substance use problems include a tendency to select actions associated with immediate gain, at the cost of long-term losses or negative future consequences, insufficient consideration of the probability and magnitude of reward of available options and a reliance on habitual behaviour. It is thought that these may reflect altered brain circuitry sub-serving decision-making processes.[10,11]

Alcohol

Many (50%–80%) individuals experiencing alcohol use disorders experience mild to moderate deficits in cognitive functioning, particularly in learning and memory, spatial ability and executive functions.[12-14] In contrast, there is a relative sparing of general intelligence and language skills. Memory deficits tend to show some recovery within weeks of abstinence, whereas executive functioning deficits have a more protracted course of recovery,[13-16] with evidence of impairment in some functions after several months of abstinence.[17-19]

Illicit drugs

In comparison to alcohol, research on cognitive impairment following prolonged/chronic drug use is in its infancy. However, over the past decade studies have found widespread impairments in the memory and executive functioning of people using amphetamines,[20] 3,4-methylenedioxymethamphetamine (MDMA),[21,22] cannabis,[23] crack cocaine,[24] and opiates,[25,26] with some detectable after months of abstinence. Impairments have been found in response inhibition, decision-making, planning and working memory depending on the extent and nature of drug used.[27-29]

Psychiatric disorders

Cognitive impairment is often present with several psychiatric disorders. In bipolar affective disorder, deficits have been found in verbal memory, attention and executive functioning,[3] although they are more selective and milder than in schizophrenia.[31,32] With obsessive–compulsive disorder, cognitive impairment tends to be subtle, averaging half a standard deviation below healthy controls.[33] In depressed patients, deficits have been found in planning, pattern and spatial recognition and working memory.[34] Poor performance on tests of verbal learning and memory has been observed among individuals experiencing panic disorder and social phobia relative to matched-controls.[35] However, of all psychiatric conditions, schizophrenia has been the focus of most neuropsychological research. Cognitive impairment is now recognised as a central and enduring characteristic of the illness.[36,37] With performance typically falling in the bottom 5th–10th percentile,[38] researchers have proposed its inclusion in future diagnostic criteria for schizophrenia in DSM-V.[39] Comprehensive reviews and meta-analyses have attempted to assimilate the vast and disparate evidence of both generalised impairment and specific impairments in processing speed, attention, declarative (verbal) memory, vigilance, working memory, executive functioning and social cognition.[37,40-42] Well-learned tasks, such as reading and mental arithmetic, are often unimpaired, whereas novel tasks requiring mental flexibility, problem-solving, planning and decision-making can be moderately to severely impaired. These deficits can have a profound impact on everyday life. One summary suggests 'given the multitude of tests that show significant impairment, clearly any specific impairment (e.g. memory or executive functioning) exists *within a more widespread reduction in general cognitive functioning.*[36]

The incidence of substance use disorder is higher in schizophrenia (up to 70%–80%)[43] than in other psychiatric disorders. With increasing evidence for cognitive impairment in schizophrenia and their impact on outcome, it is important to focus research attention on the neuropsychological functioning of individuals with mental health–substance use problems, particularly when the mental health disorder is schizophrenia. While cognitive impairment is by no means restricted to people with schizophrenia and substance use disorder, the limited research on other conditions suggest weaker and less disabling degrees of impairment. (For research findings on individuals with both affective disorders and substance use disorders *see* Carpenter and Hittner,[44] and Levy, Monzani, Stephansky, *et al.*[45])

Mental health–substance use: schizophrenia and substance use disorders

Despite the high prevalence of comorbid schizophrenia and substance use disorder and the evidence base for cognitive impairment in each condition separately, few studies have examined the nature and severity of impairment. One study[46] noted that selective attention, episodic memory and executive functioning (abstraction) deficits are shared by the two conditions, whereas visuospatial deficits and retrograde amnesia (more prominent in alcoholism), and expressive language deficits and slower reaction times (more prominent in schizophrenia) differentiate them. Since most substances achieve their reinforcing effects through the dopaminergic system,[47] which plays a key role in both cognition[48] and schizophrenia,[49] some important questions are raised concerning individuals with both conditions. Do the cognitive deficits associated with two disorders separately converge, resulting in impairment of greater severity? In other words, is there an 'additive effect'? Since there are both common and differentiating deficits, does their co-occurrence result in greater generalised cognitive impairment or is any additive effect restricted to specific cognitive domains? In addition to the neurotoxic effects of substance misuse, individuals may experience head injuries (e.g. from falls or acts of violence when intoxicated) and nutritional deficits which also affect cognitive functioning.

We now summarise the findings from studies that have made direct comparisons between people experiencing mental health–substance use and the non-substance using individual experiencing schizophrenia.

Mental health and alcohol use disorders

After nicotine, alcohol is the most widely misused substance among individuals experiencing schizophrenia,[50-52] yet relatively few studies have examined cognitive functioning in people both experiencing schizophrenia and alcohol use disorders. The first US study focusing on this population found no evidence for the additive effect on a test of executive function (set-shifting) and face recognition.[53] However, contradictory findings have emerged from three US studies[54-56] reporting greater cognitive impairment among individuals with both schizophrenia and alcohol use disorders relative to those with only schizophrenia. Two further US studies reported findings in support of the additive effect on middle-aged and elderly populations.[57,58]

In the UK, our research found that people experiencing mental health–substance use problems achieve a lower age-adjusted total Mini Mental State Examination (MMSE) score relative to individuals experiencing only schizophrenia or alcohol use disorder, but with significant item differences confined to the visual-construction item.[59] In a later study, on a battery of memory and executive functioning tests, a consistently poorer performance was observed among mental health–substance use (indicating greater global impairment) but with statistically significant differences on set-shifting, working memory, planning and delayed verbal memory.[60] Most of the studies examining comorbid alcohol use disorders point towards poorer attention, memory (including visuospatial memory) and executive functioning, in particular working memory. Although some studies have failed to find differences between mental health–substance use and schizophrenia-only groups,[61] none has reported better performance among individuals experiencing mental health–substance use problems. In summary, there appears to be evidence of greater impairment on specific cognitive domains, as well as a more global/generalised cognitive deficit among individuals with schizophrenia who also misuse alcohol.

Mental health and drug use disorders

Most research has been conducted on heterogeneous groups of people using a range of substances. The few studies that have examined or undertaken separate analyses on schizophrenia and cannabis use disorder have generated mixed findings, with little evidence in support of an additive effect.[62] Studies of comorbid cocaine use disorder are equally divergent.[63,64] With an increasing number of studies reporting equal or better executive functioning in people experiencing mental health–substance use problems, evidence for the additive effect of cocaine use disorder and schizophrenia remains weak.

In studies examining generic substance users/misusers, alcohol misuse typically represents less than one-third of the mental health–substance use population. One study failed to find general or domain specific differences on 60 neuropsychological measures between mental health–substance use (former substance abusers) and schizophrenia only experiencing individuals.[65] Similarly using comprehensive batteries, other studies have failed to find evidence in support of an additive effect.[66–69] In contrast, a number of studies have reported superior performance, particularly on measures of executive functioning (verbal fluency, set-shifting) and on measures of visuospatial memory and psychomotor speed.[70,72,73] Various explanations have been proposed for this seemingly counterintuitive finding. Some researchers suggest that the procurement of illicit drugs requires high-level executive functions such as planning, problem-solving and social skills,[74] thus higher functioning individuals are those more likely to engage in drug use. One study suggested that with their more intact executive capacity, individuals experiencing mental health–substance use problems may profit from accelerated interventions to alleviate boredom and non-compliance.[67]

Given the evidence for the additive effect of alcohol use and evidence of equivalent or superior functioning for people using illicit drugs, contradictory findings emerging from the broader literature examining heterogeneous mental health–substance use might be expected. It is possible that cognitive impairment only manifests as poor performance on neuropsychological testing, beyond a certain severity threshold, i.e. in cases of heavy and prolonged/chronic substance use. In some studies, individuals experiencing mental health–substance use problems were users rather than misusers of drugs, or only past misusers. It is likely that current misusers and substance-dependent users exhibit greater cognitive impairment. It is also possible that alcohol has a more detrimental effect on cognitive functioning than illicit drugs. A recent meta-analysis of studies examining neuropsychological functioning in individuals with schizophrenia and substance use disorders concluded that working memory deficits were exhibited among alcohol but not drug misusers.[75]

METHODOLOGICAL LIMITATIONS

There is little doubt that the contradictory findings to date are at least partially explained by methodological limitations and discrepancies across studies. Some of the methodological shortcomings include the examination of only specific neuropsychological domains, a failure to control for levels of pre-morbid functioning and shortfalls in the matching of samples (e.g. age, education and symptom severity). Others include limited sample sizes, insufficient statistical power to detect group differences and a reliance upon normative data published in different test manuals. Finally, the failure to eliminate or at least statistically control for confounds, such as medication (with better performance reported in people on atypical compared to typical antipsychotics[76]) is another limitation. Differences in sampling (e.g. inpatient versus outpatient, chronic versus acute schizophrenia, substance use versus misuse), methodology (cognitive domain examined, sensitivity of neuropsychological test and performance parameter selected), timeframe for substance disorders (e.g. current or lifetime) and timing of the assessment (i.e. length of abstinence and time-dependent recovery) each hamper direct comparisons across studies.

IDENTIFYING COGNITIVE IMPAIRMENT
Neuropsychological assessment

Cognitive deficits are not always obvious to the professional and thus the individuals' resulting behaviour may be misinterpreted as poor motivation. Increasing health professionals' awareness of cognitive deficits can enhance therapeutic rapport, for example, by increasing their sensitivity to the individual.[77] Routine screening for cognitive deficits can identify those in need of more detailed assessment or additional support in rehabilitation. The most widely and universally used screen is the Mini Mental State Examination.[78] Others include:

➤ Montreal Cognitive Assessment (MoCA)[79]
➤ Addenbrookes Cognitive Exam[80]
➤ Repeatable Battery for the Assessment of Neuropsychological Status (RBANS)[81]
➤ Kaplan-Baycrest Neuropsychological Assessment.[82]

(For guidance on suitable screening and assessment tools please refer to Lezak, Howieson and Loring;[8] Hodges;[83] and Strauss, Sherman and Spreen.[84])

Pre-morbid IQ is usually estimated from performance on standardised measures of reading ability, e.g. the National Adult Reading Test,[85] or the Wechsler Test of Adult Reading.[86] However, where individuals are dysphasic, dyslexic, or speak English only as a second language, a detailed assessment of their educational and occupational history can be used to provide a crude estimate of pre-morbid functioning.

The comprehensive evaluation of cognitive functioning should be conducted by a neuropsychologist or a clinical psychologist and usually takes the form of a standardised neuropsychological battery. It will normally include assessment of pre-morbid and current intellectual functioning (IQ), supplemented with tests measuring the specific cognitive domains of interest. Much of the research in mental health–substance use has used standardised batteries of tests designed to assess multiple cognitive functions; for example:

➤ Halstead-Reitan Neurological Test Battery[87]
➤ Neurobiological Cognitive Status Examination.[88]

More recently it has included computerised assessments such as the CANTAB.[89] Neuropsychological batteries developed specifically to assess cognitive functioning in people experiencing schizophrenia include:

➤ Brief Assessment of Cognition in Schizophrenia[90,91]
➤ MATRICS Consensus Cognitive Battery (MCCB).[92]

Self-report questionnaires

In addition to neuropsychological tests, self-report questionnaires can assist the professionals' observations of cognitive inefficiencies. Useful examples include:

➤ Cognitive Failures Questionnaire (CFQ)[93]
➤ Everyday Memory Questionnaire[94]
➤ Subjective Scale to Investigate Cognition in Schizophrenia[95]
➤ The Dysexecutive Questionnaire.[96]

BEHAVIOURS ASSOCIATED WITH COGNITIVE IMPAIRMENT

Identifying cognitive deficits in psychiatric and substance using populations poses several challenges. Deficits tend to be more subtle than those found in neurological populations and the behavioural symptoms of the psychiatric condition can mask or overlap with those resulting from cognitive failures. In addition, individuals experiencing mental health–substance use problems often demonstrate relatively intact intellectual functioning, alongside a wide range of other intact capabilities. However, executive deficits may leave them less able to initiate, organise or monitor their actions in order to obtain their goals, or less able to inhibit inappropriate dysfunctional behaviours. Poor self-regulation and poor emotional control can trigger irritability, outbursts of frustration and a general lack of patience, affecting several aspects of daily functioning. It is important to consider subjective complaints about thinking and memory problems and to be aware of certain behaviours or characteristics that can indicate underlying cognitive impairments (see Table 8.1).

TABLE 8.1 Examples of observed or reported behaviours indicative of cognitive impairment

Behaviour	Possible area of cognitive dysfunction
Constant requests to repeat information.	Attention deficits
Unable to recall knowledge or reflect on experiences of therapy, but when provided with cues or prompts they can recall some of what they were told previously.	Declarative memory (problems retrieving information)
Failing to carry out intended behaviours, e.g. attend support groups, homework.	Impaired prospective memory or executive dysfunction (impaired initiation)
Not being able to do more than one thing at a time, e.g. hold a conversation while packing up to leave.	Impaired cognitive flexibility
Difficulty retaining information while doing something with it; e.g. remembering a phone number while dialling.	Working memory
Inability to inhibit behaviours (drinking/using substances when exposed to environmental cues) even though the person reports wanting to stop this behaviour in clinic sessions.	Impaired inhibition (resulting in organic impulsivity)
Inability to anticipate consequence of events, plan or organise.	Executive deficits (e.g. impaired forward thinking, reasoning or decision-making)
A lack of verbal participation in group settings.	Language deficits (impaired verbal fluency, dysphasia) and/or memory problems (difficulty following conversation)
Problems communicating the details of a story in an organised sequential manner.	Language deficits (impaired verbal fluency, dysphasia) and/or executive deficits (impaired planning, organisation).

Observing behaviour and interaction in both one-to-one and group settings can help identify subtle but clinically important cognitive deficits.[97] Cognitive impairment is often associated with problems in employment and self-esteem, so information on the individual's day-to-day functioning and whether any restrictions/limitations relate to cognitive deficits can be informative. Their identification is important because if ignored, people with the greatest need stand to profit the least from treatment, leading to poorer outcomes and a likely reappearance in treatment. An understanding of the nature and severity of cognitive impairments and their prognostic implications can help inform diagnosis, treatment and rehabilitation planning.

THE IMPACT OF COGNITIVE IMPAIRMENTS ON PSYCHOLOGICAL INTERVENTIONS

Cognitive impairment can predict course of symptoms, treatment response, retention and compliance relapse and functional outcome.[98–100] All of these are important in the management of mental health–substance use. People treated for mental illness and substance use disorders need to learn skills for coping with symptoms and to evaluate complex information and initiate and execute plans. Impaired attention, memory and executive functioning can restrict an individual's ability to understand the treatment requirements, leading to poor attendance and compliance. For example, subtle attention and memory deficits can cause difficulties managing medication schedules and it may be necessary for professionals to adjust their instructions accordingly. A successful treatment outcome is dependent upon the use of complex cognitive functions that facilitate planning, problem-solving, memory, mental flexibility and reasoning.[101,102] These skills are fundamental for processing psychoeducational materials, engaging in psychological interventions and for sustained behavioural adaptation. Psychological interventions typically require the individual to draw on a complex system of selective and sustained attention, memory, problem-solving, reasoning and abstraction; and to apply in the real world what is learned in treatment.[101] Individuals need to reflect on their experiences, temporarily hold ideas/thoughts while focusing on others, self-monitor, and internalise the meaning of events, which places heavy demands on cognition. Cognitive behaviour therapy (CBT – *see* Book 4, Chapter 10; Book 5, Chapters 11, 12) is used to increase a person's repertoire of coping skills in resisting urges to use substances. With deficits in verbal memory, the individual experiencing mental health–substance use disorders might struggle to recall the material discussed in previous sessions. CBT assumes an ability to draw on experiences in the recent past (episodic memory), consider situations from multiple/different perspectives (mental flexibility) apply abstract concepts and principles to future behaviours (planning and organisation) and respond appropriately, while processing information in an organised and rational way. The setting of homework, for example, may be difficult for people with marked memory and planning deficits. Relapse prevention[103] (*see* Book 6, Chapters 15, 16) assumes the individual has intact executive functioning to enable them to identify signs of relapse and initiate strategies to avoid or manage them effectively. Even where strategies to manage situations (e.g. auditory hallucinations) are in place, poor memory or initiation may impede their execution. Similarly, motivational interviewing (*see* Book 4, Chapter 7) requires the individual to weigh up pros and cons and identify future goals, thus placing heavy demands on declarative and working memory, mental flexibility, planning and abstraction. For people experiencing mental health–substance use disorders, any programme reliant on the storage of large amounts of verbal information or mental flexibility may have limited application.

THE MODIFICATION OF PSYCHOLOGICAL INTERVENTIONS

Recent controlled trials suggest that integrated programmes that take into consideration cognitive and motivational deficits (*see* Book 5, Chapter 11) yield the most promise, with significant reductions in hospitalisations, homelessness, unemployment and substance use.[104,105] Modifications to motivational interviewing techniques to accommodate cognitive deficits and disordered thinking have been proposed.[106,107] These include the use of repetition, simplifying open-ended questions, refining reflective listening skills and heightening emphasis on affirmation. They also advocate active reflection and summarising to promote cognitive organisation and a reliance on concrete language and short-term goals.

With evidence of both global and specific memory and reasoning impairments, one study[108] made recommendations on how treatment programmes can be modified for individuals experiencing mental health–substance use disorders. The authors suggest that prior to making any adjustments, one considers the individual's potential for learning and change, their level of awareness of deficits (insight), psychological and personality variables, duration and severity of psychiatric and substance use symptoms. For moderate to severe cognitive impairment, professionals should reduce the rate, amount, duration and complexity of information presented. Interactive, repetitive approaches with reliance on verbal paradigms initially are encouraged, whereas those heavily reliant on memory processes and abstract thinking should be kept to a minimum. Similarly, treatment components relying on higher-order skills (e.g. relapse prevention) may require more gradual introduction, when time-dependent recovery following abstinence is likely to have occurred. The following section outlines some ways in which treatment can be adapted to accommodate specific cognitive deficits frequently seen in individuals experiencing mental health–substance use disorders. It is important to stress that these techniques have proven useful in clinical practice with individuals who have acquired brain injury, but their effectiveness on mental health–substance use populations has not been empirically tested. However, enhancing treatment compliance is of paramount importance with such individuals, and any technique that optimises attention, retention and recall is likely to be a step in the right direction.

WORKING WITH DEFICITS IN ATTENTION

Attention (ability to detect, react, select, sustain, shift between and mentally track stimuli or information) is a fundamental requirement to any treatment intervention. People with attention deficits are likely to benefit from more structured treatment delivered in shorter, more frequent sessions, to avoid 'overloading'. Limit the amount of auditory information presented and supplement with written forms (e.g. handouts). This will aid processing during the session and facilitate learning between sessions. The pace of delivery should be reduced, for example, chunking information into semantically related sections, use of cue cards and providing regular breaks. Information must be made as interesting, relevant and as enjoyable as possible to optimise attention and consolidation of information. One study recommend using humour, anecdotes, voice intonation changes, colour and visual aids.[109] Where treatment is delivered in group settings, group member size should be kept to a minimum to avoid distractions. Therapeutic sessions are most effective when conducted in a quiet room, free from disturbances and interruptions and with minimal competing stimuli in the surrounding environment. While individuals experiencing mental health–substance use disorders often demonstrate preserved verbal skills, in cases where receptive language impairments are identified, use short sentences, high-frequency words and simple jargon-free language, using pictorial communication aids wherever possible.

WORKING WITH DEFICITS IN LEARNING AND MEMORY

To accommodate memory and learning deficits, use of repetition, frequent summaries and session revisions are encouraged.[110] Our own research suggested that people experiencing mental health–substance use disorders experience problems retrieving/accessing stored information rather than problems encoding information, and that rehearsal (repetition) and prompts improve recall.[60] In practice this means important messages to be conveyed (e.g. medication instructions) may require multiple presentations, offering the opportunity for rehearsal, along with simplified written instructions to aid clarity (e.g. in bullet point form). One study[108] recommends the use of mnemonics (i.e. first letter cueing via making rhymes), categorising, chunking and visual imagery. It is important to understand the nature of the individual's deficit and to adopt mediums that draw on their relative cognitive strengths. For example, conveying information in a visual form, such as film, drawings, illustrations, when marked verbal memory deficits are present. For the more severely impaired, environmental modifications can be made to reduce demands on memory, for example, signposts, labels, wall charts, planners or checklists. Individuals should be encouraged to adopt highly structured daily routines that facilitate repetition, where implicit learning can play a greater role. Compensatory memory aids, e.g. diaries, audiotapes or videotapes of sessions, and electronic organisers, such as computers, watches, mobile phones and the like with alarms programmed to generate reminders are widely used with brain-injured patients.[111,112] Finally, carers or family members should be encouraged to use repetition, and can be enlisted as co-therapists to facilitate between-session learning and prompt homework completion.[4,113]

WORKING WITH DEFICITS IN EXECUTIVE FUNCTIONING

Impaired working memory, mental flexibility, planning and organisational skills can cause difficulties holding long term consequences in mind and can impede ability to switch ideas, generalise and think creatively. Essentially, they are skills that enable people to cope with many real-life situations.[114] However, because executive problems are multidimensional there cannot be a single treatment approach; rather interventions should be considered in relation to the presenting problem area.

Managing impulsivity/disinhibition

Substance use may offer a more immediate but maladaptive means of combating symptoms such as auditory hallucinations, or social isolation.[115] It is thought that substance misuse is determined by automatic processes and that an ability to override such behaviours relies heavily on the integrity of executive processes.[116] It is, therefore, important when working with impulsive/disinhibited individuals to encourage self-monitoring, self-regulation and planning, as the disinhibiting effects of substances can lead to risky behaviours, such as sexual promiscuity or engagement in criminal activities.

It is important to set up self-monitoring training to help reduce impulsive responses (e.g. substance use – *see* Book 4, Chapter 13), and to utilise a goal-setting system to help direct behaviour towards the desired outcome of abstinence. Maintaining abstinence requires an inhibition of automatic responses (e.g. to craving cues) and the shifting of attention (e.g. thoughts of craving) to alternative behaviours which may be complicated by the presence of competing distractions (e.g. hallucinations). Self-questioning, revising personal goals, reflecting on the pros and cons of behaviours and predicting likely outcomes can help diffuse situations of intense craving. Asking individuals to imagine facing the temptation to use substances in different situations and giving examples of when their coping strategy might fail (probing for alternatives/back-ups) can be helpful. Verbalising and practising responses in high-risk situations, using role play to rehearse refusal skills, increase the likelihood of such strategies being used. To increase skill generalisation and use of coping strategies in novel situations use simple rules and multiple realistic examples, for best effect. Cue cards with key words to prompt the use of strategies, e.g. 'stop, think, check', can be given to individuals to carry in their wallets. Impulsivity and disinhibition can also cause problems in the management of behaviour during therapeutic interactions. Explicitly defining the therapeutic relationship (*see* Book 4, Chapter 2) and its boundaries, for example, by drawing up behavioural contracts that state the consequences of an agreement breach, can help with over-familiarity and inappropriate behaviour. Finally, relaxation or mindfulness techniques may be taught to help diffuse emotions states such as anger, which would otherwise obstruct the therapeutic rapport.

Managing initiation, planning and mental flexibility deficits

Expressive language, semantic or phonemic fluency deficits may leave the individual unable to articulate their thoughts or feelings, leading to frustration. Individuals may benefit from a more directive therapeutic style, e.g. with professionals providing alternatives to maladaptive thoughts and behaviours.[117] In the learning disability/brain injury field, minimising open-ended questions, using written mind-mapping techniques, diagrams, neuroimaging scans and checklists can help cement information and ideas with individuals with limited cognitive flexibility.[113] Deficits in planning and initiation are likely to influence both attendance and contribution at therapeutic sessions. Teaching 'step-by-step' problem-solving approaches, for example, goal ladders delineating short- and long-term goals and how these are to be achieved by subdividing into smaller, more manageable tasks can help the person organise ideas and priorities.[117] Essentially, individuals should be encouraged to carry out the following steps:

1 Identify the problem.
2 Set measurable, realistic and concrete goals.
3 Generate solutions.
4 Monitor attempts/success.[108]

Adapting to new situations (e.g. a life no longer centred around substance use) requires careful treatment planning and long-term support and encouragement. Individuals should be encouraged to rehearse newly learned problem-solving strategies to deal with everyday problems that arise. Health professionals can reinforce strategies with coaching (e.g. weekly reviews of progress) and supervision until the skills are consolidated and firmly acquired. Box 8.1 offers some tips for therapeutic sessions/general management.

BOX 8.1 Tips for therapeutic sessions/general management

Attention, memory and learning

- Keep sessions short and frequent.
- Include booster sessions.
- Minimise distractions.
- Have regular breaks.
- Limit amount of information presented (avoid overload).
- Use repetition and rehearsal.
- Use summaries and reviews and checklists.
- Use multiple sensory modalities (auditory, written, pictorial).
- Include reading material to improve attention, comprehension and retention of information.
- Make information interesting, relevant and enjoyable.
- Use humour and voice intonations.
- Use simple language.
- Avoid jargon.
- Use diagrams, illustrations, film, or cartoons to compensate for verbal memory deficits.
- Encourage compensatory aids, e.g. diaries, filofaxes, calendars, electronic organisers, mobile phones, and so forth, to act as prospective memory aids.

Executive dysfunction

- Use relaxation techniques to dampen arousal states (e.g. anger, impulsivity).
- Use simple rules and real-life examples to aid problems with abstract thinking.
- Challenge the individual's contributions and encourage the generation of alternatives.
- Adopt a more directive therapeutic style.
- Ask guided questions that elicit solutions when they fail to initiate any spontaneously.
- Set clear boundaries.
- Subdivide goals into smaller tasks.
- Facilitate self-monitoring by teaching strategies such as 'stop, think, check' before acting impulsively.
- Use role play to practise strategies for coping/managing triggers, and relapse, symptoms.
- Encourage individuals to (1) identify the problem; (2) set measurable, realistic goals; (3) generate solutions; and (4) monitor attempts/success.

PROVIDING FEEDBACK

Neuropsychologists typically provide feedback on cognitive performance in the context of the individual's cognitive strengths and weaknesses. With multiple relapses and treatment episodes people experiencing mental health–substance use disorders may internalise their failures as personal flaws, leading to feelings of hopelessness and diminishing motivation to engage in future attempts. Providing an explanation for some of their areas of difficulty, and how their cognitive strengths can compensate for their weaknesses forms an important part of the rehabilitation process. Externalising difficulties as symptoms of their illness, rather than underlying personality traits resistant to change, can enhance self-efficacy. Finally, discussion about the research evidence for recovery from cognitive impairment with increasing periods of abstinence can be highly motivating.

COGNITIVE REHABILITATION IN MENTAL HEALTH–SUBSTANCE USE: WHAT DOES THE FUTURE HOLD?

Cognitive remediation

The limited longitudinal research on the course of cognitive impairment in the individual experiencing mental health–substance use disorders suggests that without intervention (e.g. cessation of substance misuse), it remains relatively stable over time.[118,119] Since cognitive impairment is associated with poor compliance and self-efficacy, its rehabilitation is likely to facilitate gains in multiple areas of functioning. Cognitive remediation assumes that the process of brain plasticity (the idea that it is capable of changing its structure and function, reorganising and adapting) can be aided by stimulating the brain functions associated with the area of deficit. Stimulation usually entails repetitively practising tasks that require the cognitive skill. The theoretical assumption is that any improvement will generalise to everyday functioning, e.g. social behaviour, work and employment. There are a number of cognitive remediation programmes available including Neurocognitive Enhancement Therapy[120] and the Neuropsychological Educational Approach to Remediation (NEAR).[121]

Cognitive remediation has been investigated in people experiencing schizophrenia, who have shown improvement on the tasks they were trained to complete.[122–124] Cognitive Remediation Therapy (CRT)[125] was designed for people experiencing schizophrenia and has been subjected to the most rigorous empirical testing.[126] It explicitly teaches and practises thinking skills aimed at rehabilitating attention, memory and executive functioning deficits and relies heavily on didactic training. It is tailored to the individual's cognitive capacity, with graduated increases in difficulty to facilitate errorless learning.[127] Improvements in neuropsychological functioning have been detected up to 6 months following 12 weeks (40 hours) of CRT.[128] However, a Cochrane review concludes that the evidence for the effectiveness of CRT is inconclusive.[129] The primary limitation is the paucity of evidence that improvement on neuropsychological testing generalises to everyday functioning. While a promising area for future research, all of the CRT studies to date have excluded comorbid substance users, and thus there is no evidence supporting its application in mental health–substance use disorder. Furthermore, given the intensity of CRT (i.e. several sessions per week over the course of a few months), programme adherence may be a particular challenge for individuals experiencing mental health–substance use problems.

THE ROLE OF NEW TECHNOLOGIES

New technologies are emerging all the time, offering dynamic and flexible methods of treatment delivery and as compensatory aids. For example, DVDs and e-learning programmes have increased access to psychological therapies and computer-based modular approaches enable an individual to work at his/her own pace. Digitally portable media, e.g. podcasts, offer an alternative to traditional learning methods for individuals with good/preserved auditory memory. While there are no evaluations on the use of such technologies with cognitively impaired individuals experiencing mental health–substance use disorders, it is plausible that they will enhance functional outcomes by strengthening learning skills. Virtual reality games enlist visuospatial skills, strategy generation, planning skills and coordination and offer rehabilitative potential to practise skills for independent living, e.g. shopping, and have been used with people experiencing schizophrenia.[130] Similarly, interactive home video game consoles (e.g. Nintendo Wii) heavily reliant on physical activity may improve hand–eye coordination, visuospatial, planning and organisation skills; this is a desirable outcome for people taking antipsychotic medication associated with weight gain.

PHARMACOLOGICAL TREATMENTS

Increasing evidence in support of the impact on cognitive impairment on treatment has stimulated efforts to find pharmacological agents to enhance cognitive functioning (*see* Book 5, Chapter 13). While drugs exist for the treatment of degenerative brain diseases such as Alzheimer's (e.g. donepezil, rivastigmine, galantamine), agents to improve mild to moderate deficits in psychiatric and substance-using populations are not yet established. Early findings suggest that modafinil can improve executive functioning, attention and motor performance in people experiencing schizophrenia,[131] though it may be ineffective with people receiving antipsychotic medications.[132] Clinical trials of the neurosteroid pregnenolone are currently taking place among schizophrenia populations,[133] and if effective may warrant future investigation with those experiencing mental health–substance use disorders.

THE NEED FOR ONGOING SUPPORT AND SOCIALISATION

For people recently discharged from hospital or supported accommodation, the challenges of returning to independent living can be amplified where there is cognitive impairment. Cognitive functioning is associated with service use,[134] and degree of social support necessary to maintain an outpatient status.[135] Although severe mental illness is characterised by isolation, recent studies on mental health–substance use report evidence of better social competence. This has been coined the 'paradox of the dually diagnosed'.[136] Actively engaging in community activities provides a structure to one's day and increases socialisation and social capital. Rehabilitation has been described as '*a process where people who are disabled by injury or disease work together with professional staff, relatives and members of the wider community to achieve their optimum physical, psychological, social and vocational wellbeing*.[137] People experiencing mental health–substance use disorders should be encouraged to engage in activities that promote healthy lifestyles (e.g. sports and exercise) that also serve to improve social reintegration and quality of life. Finally, exposure to positive role models by attending mutual self-help recovery groups may offer additional support and socialisation.

CONCLUSION

The literature suggests that individuals experiencing mental health–substance use disorders, particularly schizophrenia and alcohol misuse, experience significant impairments in attention, memory and executive deficits. There is weaker evidence of an additive effect of illicit drug use on the already compromised cognitive functioning in people experiencing schizophrenia. Understanding the nature and severity of cognitive impairments in mental health–substance use, as well as their prognostic implications, can help inform diagnosis, treatment and rehabilitation planning. It is likely that these individuals with the greatest need will profit the least from treatment, without modifications that capitalise on cognitive strengths and accommodate cognitive deficits. Longitudinal research is needed to determine the recovery of impaired cognitive functioning during periods of prolonged abstinence. Future research should examine the effectiveness of cognitive rehabilitation as a means of enhancing treatment engagement, retention and response. However, it is possible that a combined approach of cognitive remediation, intervention modification and pharmacotherapy could offer the most effective means of improving outcomes among cognitively impaired individuals experiencing mental health–substance use problems.

REFERENCES

1 Cleary M, Hunt GE, Matheson S, *et al*. Views of Australian mental health stakeholders on clients' problematic drug and alcohol use. *Drug and Alcohol Review*. 2009; **28**: 122–8.

2 Kastrup M. Who became revolving door patients? Findings from a nation-wide cohort of first time admitted psychiatric patients. *Acta Psychiatrica Scandinavica*. 1987; **76**: 80–8.

3 Ziedonis D, Trudeau K. Motivation to quit using substances among individuals with schizophrenia: implications for a motivation-based treatment model. *Schizophrenia Bulletin*. 1997; **23**: 229–38.

4 Blume AW, Davis JM, Schmaling KB. Neurocognitive dysfunction in dually diagnosed patients: a potential roadblock to motivating behavior change. *Journal of Psychoactive Drugs*. 1999; **31**: 111–15.

5 Harrison C, Abou-Saleh MT. Psychiatric disorders and substance misuse psychopathology. In: Rassool GH, editor. *Dual Diagnosis: substance misuse and psychiatric disorders*. Oxford: Blackwell; 2002.

6 Reber AS, Reber E, editors. *Dictionary of Psychology*. 3rd ed. St Ives: Penguin Books; 2001.

7 Baddeley AD. *Human Memory: theory and practice*. Revised edition. Hove: Psychology Press; 1997.

8 Lezak MD, Howieson DB, Loring DW. *Neuropsychological Assessment*. 4th ed. New York: Oxford University Press; 2004.

9 Volkow ND, Fowler JS, Wang GJ. The addicted human brain viewed in the light of imaging studies: brain circuits and treatment strategies. *Neuropharmacology*. 2004; **47**: 3–13.

10 Bechara A, Damasio H. Decision-making and addiction (part I): impaired activation of

somatic states in substance dependent individuals when pondering decisions with negative future consequences. *Neuropsychologia*. 2002; **40**: 1675–89.

11 Fishbein DH, Eldreth DLM, Hyde C, *et al*. Risky decision making and the anterior cingulate cortex in abstinent drug abusers and nonusers. *Cognitive Brain Research*. 2005; **23**: 119–36.

12 Bates ME, Bowden SC, Barry D. Neurocognitive impairment associated with alcohol use disorders: implications for treatment. *Experimental and Clinical Psychopharmacology*. 2002; **10**: 193–212.

13 Zinn S, Stein R, Swartzwelder HS. Executive functioning early in abstinence from alcohol. *Alcohol Clinical and Experimental Research*. 2004; **28**: 1338–46.

14 Scheurich A. Neuropsychological functioning and alcohol dependence. *Current Opinion in Psychiatry*. 2005; **18**: 319–23.

15 Mann K, Gunther A, Stetter F, *et al*. Rapid recovery from cognitive deficits in abstinent alcoholics: a controlled test-retest study. *Alcohol and Alcoholism*. 1999; **34**: 567–74.

16 Manning V, Wanigaratne S, Best D, *et al*. Changes in neuropsychological functioning during alcohol detoxification. *European Addiction Research*. 2008; **14**: 226–33.

17 Munro CA, Saxton J, Butters MA. The neuropsychological consequences of abstinence among older alcoholics: a cross-sectional study. *Alcohol: Clinical and Experimental Research*. 2000; **24**: 1510–16.

18 Davies SJ, Pandit SA, Feeney A, *et al*. Is there cognitive impairment in clinically 'healthy' abstinent alcohol dependence? *Alcohol and Alcoholism*. 2005; **40**: 498–503.

19 Rourke SB, Grant I. The interactive effects of age and length of abstinence on the recovery of neuropsychological functioning in chronic male alcoholics: a 2-year follow-up study. *Journal of the International Neuropsychological Society*. 1999; **5**: 234–46.

20 Ornstein TJ, Iddon JL, Baldacchino AM, *et al*. Profiles of cognitive dysfunction in chronic amphetamine and heroin abusers. *Neuropsychopharmacology*. 2000; **23**: 113–26.

21 Kalechstein AD, De La Garza R, Mahoney JJ, *et al*. MDMA use and neurocognition: a meta-analytic review. *Psychopharmacology (Berl)*. 2007; **189**: 531–7.

22 Ersche KD, Clark L, London M, *et al*. Profile of executive and memory function associated with amphetamine and opiate dependence. *Neuropsychopharmacology*. 2006; **31**: 1036–47.

23 Solowij N, Stephens RS, Roffman RA, *et al*. Cognitive functioning of long-term heavy cannabis users seeking treatment. *Journal of the American Medical Association*. 2002; **287**: 1123–31.

24 Di Sclafani V, Tolou-Shams M, Price LJ, *et al*. Neuropsychological performance of individuals dependent on crack-cocaine, or crack-cocaine and alcohol, at 6 weeks and 6 months of abstinence. *Drug Alcohol Dependence*. 2002; **66**: 161–71.

25 Davis PE, Liddiard H, McMillan TM. Neuropsychological deficits and opiate abuse. *Drug Alcohol Dependence*. 2002; **67**: 105–8.

26 Mintzer MZ, Copersino ML, Stitzer ML. Opioid abuse and cognitive performance. *Drug Alcohol Dependence*. 2005; **78**: 225–30.

27 Rogers RD, Robbins TW. The neuropsychology of chronic drug abuse. In: Ron MA, Robbins TW, editors. *Disorders of Brain and Mind*. Cambridge: Cambridge University Press; 2003.

28 Verdejo-Garcia A, Lopez-Torrecillas F, Gimenez CO, *et al*. Clinical implications and methodological challenges in the study of the neuropsychological correlates of cannabis, stimulant, and opioid abuse. *Neuropsychological Review*. 2004; **14**: 1–41.

29 Ersche KD, Sahakian BJ. The neuropsychology of amphetamine and opiate dependence: implications for treatment. *Neuropsychological Review*. 2007; **17**: 317–36.

30 Arts B, Jabben N, Krabbendam L, *et al*. Meta-analyses of cognitive functioning in euthymic bipolar patients and their first-degree relatives. *Psychological Medicine*. 2008; **38**: 771–85.

31 Seidman LJ, Kremen WS, Koren D, *et al*. A comparative profile analysis of neuropsychological functioning in patients with schizophrenia and bipolar psychoses *Schizophrenia Research*. 2002; **53**: 31–44.

32 Toulopoulou T, Quraishi S, McDonald C, *et al*. The Maudsley Family Study: premorbid and current general intellectual function levels in familial bipolar I disorder and schizophrenia. *Journal of Clinical and Experimental Neuropsychology*. 2006; **28**: 243–59.

33 Burdick KE, Robinson DG, Malhotra AK, *et al*. Neurocognitive profile analysis in obsessive-compulsive disorder. *Journal of the International Neuropsychological Society*. 2008; **14**: 640–5.

34 Elliott R, Sahakian BJ, McKay AP, *et al*. Neuropsychological impairments in unipolar depression: the influence of perceived failure on subsequent performance. *Psychological Medicine*. 1996; **26**: 975–90.

35 Asmundson GJ, Stein MB, Larsen DK, *et al*. Neurocognitive function in panic disorder and social phobia patients. *Anxiety*. 1994; **1**: 201–7.

36 O'Carroll R. Cognitive impairment in schizophrenia. *Advances in Psychiatric Treatment*. 2000; **6**: 161–8.

37 Hoff AL, Kremen WS. Neuropsychology in schizophrenia: an update. *Current Opinion in Psychiatry*. 2003; **16**: 149–55.

38 Keefe RS. Cognitive deficits in patients with schizophrenia: effects and treatment. *Journal of Clinical Psychiatry*. 2007; **68**: 8–13.

39 Keefe RS, Fenton WS. How should DSM-V criteria for schizophrenia include cognitive impairment? *Schizophrenia Bulletin*. 2007; **33**: 912–20.

40 Heinrichs R, Zakzanis KK. Neurocognitive deficit in schizophrenia: a quantitative review of the evidence. *Neuropsychology*. 1998; **12**: 426–45.

41 Nuechterlein KH, Barch DM, Gold JM, *et al*. Identification of separable cognitive factors in schizophrenia. *Schizophrenia Research*. 2004; **72**: 29–39.

42 Johnson-Selfridge M, Zalewski C. Moderator variables of executive functioning in schizophrenia: meta-analytic findings. *Schizophrenia Bulletin*. 2001; **27**: 305–16.

43 Westermeyer J. Comorbid schizophrenia and substance abuse: a review of epidemiology and course. *American Journal of Addiction*. 2006; **15**: 345–55.

44 Carpenter KM, Hittner JB. Cognitive impairment among the dually-diagnosed: substance use history and depressive symptom correlates. *Addiction*. 1997; **92**: 747–59.

45 Levy B, Monzani BA, Stephansky MR, *et al*. Neurocognitive impairment in patients with co-occurring bipolar disorder and alcohol dependence upon discharge from inpatient care. *Psychiatry Research*. 2008; **161**: 28–35.

46 Tracy JI, Josiassen RC, Bellack AS. Neuropsychology of dual diagnosis: understanding the combined effects of schizophrenia and substance use disorders. *Clinical Psychology Review*. 1995; **15**: 67–97.

47 Kalivas PW, Volkow ND. The neural basis of addiction: a pathology of motivation and choice. *American Journal of Psychiatry*. 2005; **162**: 1403–13.

48 Remy P, Sampson Y. The role of dopamine in cognition: evidence from functional imaging studies. *Current Opinion Neurology*. 2003; **16**: 37–41.

49 Murray RM, Lappin J, Di Forti M. Schizophrenia: from developmental deviance to dopamine dysregulation. *European Neuropsychopharmacology*. 2008; **18**(Suppl. 3): S129–34.

50 Cantor-Graae E, Nordström LG, McNeil TF. Substance abuse in schizophrenia: a review of the literature and a study of correlates in Sweden. *Schizophrenia Research*. 2001; **48**: 69–82.

51 Manning V, Strathdee G, Best D, *et al*. Dual diagnosis screening: preliminary findings

on the comparison of 50 clients attending community mental health services and 50 clients attending community substance misuse services. *Journal of Substance Use*. 2002; **7**: 221–8.

52 Miles H, Johnson S, Amponsah-Afuwape S, *et al*. Characteristics of subgroups of individuals with psychotic illness and a comorbid substance use disorder. *Psychiatric Services*. 2003; **54**: 554–61.

53 Nixon SJ, Hallford HG, Tivis RD. Neurocognitive function in alcoholic, schizophrenic, and dually diagnosed patients. *Psychiatry Research*. 1996; **64**: 35–45.

54 Allen DN, Goldstein G, Aldarondo F. Neurocognitive dysfunction in patients diagnosed with schizophrenia and alcoholism. *Neuropsychology*. 1999; **13**: 62–8.

55 Allen DN, Goldstein G, Forman SD, *et al*. Neurologic examination abnormalities in schizophrenia with and without a history of alcoholism. *Neuropsychiatry, Neuropsychology and Behavioral Neurology*. 2000; **13**: 184–7.

56 Allen DN, Remy CJ. Neuropsychological deficits in patients with schizophrenia and alcohol dependence. *Archives of Clinical Neuropsychology*. 2001; **15**: 653–85.

57 Bowie CR, Serper MR, Riggio S, *et al*. Neurocognition, symptomatology, and functional skills in older alcohol-abusing schizophrenia patients. *Schizophrenia Bulletin*. 2005; **31**: 175–82.

58 Mohamed S, Bondi MW, Kasckow JW, *et al*. Neurocognitive functioning in dually diagnosed middle aged and elderly patients with alcoholism and schizophrenia. *International Journal of Geriatric Psychiatry*. 2006; **21**: 711–18.

59 Manning V, Wanigaratne S, Best D, *et al*. Screening for cognitive functioning in psychiatric outpatients with schizophrenia, alcohol dependence, and dual diagnosis. *Schizophrenia Research*. 2007; **91**: 151–8.

60 Manning V, Betteridge S, Wanigaratne S, *et al*. Cognitive impairment in dual diagnosis inpatients with schizophrenia and alcohol use disorder. *Schizophrenia Research*. 2009; **114**: 98–104.

61 Thoma P, Wiebel B, Daum I. Response inhibition and cognitive flexibility in schizophrenia with and without comorbid substance use disorder. *Schizophrenia Research*. 2007; **92**: 168–80.

62 Coulston CM, Perdices M, Tennant CC. The neuropsychological correlates of cannabis use in schizophrenia: lifetime abuse/dependence, frequency of use, and recency of use. *Schizophrenia Research*. 2007; **96**: 169–84.

63 Cooper L, Liberman D, Tucker D, *et al*. Neurocognitive deficits in the dually diagnosed with schizophrenia and cocaine abuse. *Psychiatric Rehabilitation Skills*. 1999; **3**: 231–45.

64 Serper MR, Copersino ML, Richarme D, *et al*. Neurocognitive functioning in recently abstinent, cocaine-abusing schizophrenic patients. *Journal of Substance Abuse*. 2000; **11**: 205–13.

65 Addington J, Addington D. Attentional vulnerability indicators in schizophrenia and bipolar disorder. *Schizophrenia Research*. 1997; **23**: 197–204.

66 Barnes TRE, Mutsatsa SH, Hutton SB, *et al*. Comorbid substance use and age at onset of schizophrenia. *British Journal of Psychiatry*. 2006; **188**: 237–42.

67 Herman M. Neurocognitive functioning and quality of life among dually diagnosed and non-substance abusing schizophrenia inpatients. *International Journal of Mental Health Nursing*. 2004; **13**: 282–91.

68 Wobrock T, Sittinger H, Behrendt B, *et al*. Comorbid substance abuse and neurocognitive function in recent-onset schizophrenia. *European Archives in Psychiatry and Clinical Neuroscience*. 2007; **257**: 203–10.

69 Carey KB, Carey MP, Simons JS. Correlates of substance use disorder among psychiatric outpatients: focus on cognition, social role functioning, and psychiatric status. *Journal of Nervous and Mental Disease*. 2003; **191**: 300–8.

70 Joyal CC, Halle P, Lapierre D, *et al.* Drug abuse and/or dependence and better neuropsychological performance in patients with schizophrenia. *Schizophrenia Research*. 2003; **63**: 297–9.

71 McCleery A, Addington J, Addington D. Substance misuse and cognitive functioning in early psychosis: a 2 year follow-up. *Schizophrenia Research*. 2006; **88**: 187–91.

72 Potvin S, Briand C, Prouteau A, *et al.* CANTAB explicit memory is less impaired in addicted schizophrenia patients. *Brain and Cognition*. 2005; **59**: 38–42.

73 Sevy S, Robinson DG, Holloway S, *et al.* Correlates of substance misuse in patients with first-episode schizophrenia and schizoaffective disorder. *Acta Psychiatrica Scandinavica*. 2001; **104**: 367–74.

74 Salyers MP, Mueser KT. Social functioning, psychopathology, and medication side effects in relation to substance use and abuse in schizophrenia. *Schizophrenia Research*. 2001; **48**: 109–23.

75 Potvin S, Joyal CC, Pelletier J, Stip E. Contradictory cognitive capacities among substance-abusing patients with schizophrenia: a meta-analysis. *Schizophrenia Research*. 2008; **100**: 242–51.

76 Keefe RS, Silva SG, Perkins DO, *et al.* The effects of atypical antipsychotic drugs on neurocognitive impairment in schizophrenia: a review and meta-analysis. *Schizophrenia Bulletin*. 1999; **25**: 201–22.

77 Gillen RW, Kranzler HR, Kadden RM, *et al.* Utility of a brief cognitive screening instrument in substance abuse patients: initial investigation. *Journal of Substance Abuse Treatment*. 1991; **8**: 247–51.

78 Folstein MF, Folstein SE, McHugh PR. 'Mini-mental state'. A practical method for grading the cognitive state of patients for the clinician. *Journal of Psychiatric Research*. 1975; **12**: 189–98.

79 Nasreddine ZS, Phillips NA, Bedirian V, *et al.* The Montreal Cognitive Assessment, MoCA: a brief screening tool for mild cognitive impairment. *Journal of the American Geriatric Society*. 2005; **53**: 695–9.

80 Mioshi E, Dawson K, Mitchell J, *et al.* The Addenbrooke's Cognitive Examination Revised (ACE-R): a brief cognitive test battery for dementia screening. *International Journal of Geriatric Psychiatry*. 2006; **21**: 1078–85.

81 Randolph C, Tierney MC, Mohr E, *et al.* The Repeatable Battery for the Assessment of Neuropsychological Status (RBANS): preliminary clinical validity. *Journal of Clinical and Experimental Neuropsychology*. 1998; **20**: 310–9.

82 Leach L, Kaplan E, Rewilak D, *et al. Kaplan Baycrest Neurocognitive Assessment*. San Antonio, TX: Psychological Corporation; 2000.

83 Hodges JR. *Cognitive Assessment for Clinicians*. Oxford: Oxford University Press; 1994.

84 Strauss E, Sherman E, Spreen O. *A Compendium of Neuropsychological Tests: administration, norms and commentary*. 3rd ed. New York: Oxford University Press; 2006.

85 Nelson HE, Willison JR. *NART Test Manual (part II)*. Windsor: NEFR-Nelson; 1991.

86 Wechsler D. *Wechsler Test of Adult Reading (WTAR)*. San Antonio, TX: Psychological Corporation; 2001.

87 Reitan RM, Wolfson D. *The Halstead–Reitan Neuropsychological Test Battery: theory and clinical interpretation*. 2nd ed. Tucson, AZ: Neuropsychology Press; 1993.

88 Kiernan RJ, Mueller J, Langston JW, *et al.* The Neurobehavioral Cognitive Status Examination:

a brief but quantitative approach to cognitive assessment. *Annals of Internal Medicine.* 1987; **107**: 481–5.

89 CANTAB. *Cambridge Neuropsychological Test Automated Battery.* Cambridge: Commercial Source CeNeS; 1999.

90 Keefe RS, Goldberg TE, Harvey PD, *et al.* The brief assessment of cognition in schizophrenia: reliability, sensitivity, and comparison with a standard neurocognitive battery. *Schizophrenia Research.* 2004; **68**: 283–97.

91 Keefe RS, Harvey PD, Goldberg TE, *et al.* Norms and standardization of the Brief Assessment of Cognition in Schizophrenia (BACS). *Schizophrenia Research.* 2008; **102**: 108–15.

92 Nuechterlein KH, Green MF. *MATRICS Consensus Cognitive Battery.* Los Angeles, CA: MATRICS Assessment, Inc; 2006.

93 Broadbent DE, Cooper PF, FitzGerald P, *et al.* The Cognitive Failures Questionnaire (CFQ) and its correlates. *British Journal of Clinical Psychology.* 1982; **21**: 1–16.

94 Martin M. Cognitive failure: everyday and laboratory performance. *Bulletin of the Psychonomic Society.* 1983; **21**: 97–100.

95 Stip E, Caron J, Renaud S, *et al.* Exploring cognitive complaints in schizophrenia: the subjective scale to investigate cognition in schizophrenia. *Comprehensive Psychiatry.* 2003; **44**: 331–40.

96 Burgess PW, Alderman N, Evans J, *et al.* The ecological validity of tests of executive function. *Journal of the International Neuropsychology Society.* 1998; **4**: 547–58.

97 Wilson BA. Theoretical approaches to cognitive rehabilitation. In: Goldstein LH, McNeil J, editors. *Clinical Neuropsychology: a guide to assessment and management for clinicians.* Chichester: Wiley; 2004.

98 Green MF, Kern RS, Braff DL, *et al.* Neurocognitive deficits and functional outcome in schizophrenia: are we measuring the 'right stuff'? *Schizophrenia Bulletin.* 2000; **26**: 119–36.

99 Velligan DI, Bow-Thomas CC, Mahurin RK, *et al.* Do specific neurocognitive deficits predict specific domains of community function in schizophrenia? *Journal of Nervous and Mental Disorders.* 2000; **188**: 518–24.

100 Ritsner MS. Predicting quality of life impairment in chronic schizophrenia from cognitive variables. *Quality of Life Research.* 2007; **16**: 929–37.

101 McCrady BS, Smith DE. Implications of cognitive impairment for the treatment of alcoholism. *Alcohol: Clinical and Experimental Research.* 1986; **10**: 145–9.

102 Weinstein CS, Shaffer JH. Neurocognitive aspects of substance abuse treatment: a psychotherapist's primer. *Psychotherapy.* 1993; **30**: 317–33.

103 Marlatt GA, Gordon JR. *Relapse Prevention: maintenance strategies in the treatment of addictive behaviors.* New York: Guilford Press; 1985.

104 Xie H, McHugo GJ, Helmstetter BS, *et al.* Three-year recovery outcomes for long-term patients with co-occurring schizophrenic and substance use disorders. *Schizophrenia Research.* 2005; **75**: 337–48.

105 Barrowclough C, Haddock G, Tarrier N, *et al.* Randomized controlled trial of motivational interviewing, cognitive behavior therapy, and family intervention for patients with comorbid schizophrenia and substance use disorders. *American Journal of Psychiatry.* 2001; **158**: 1706–12.

106 Martino S, Carroll K, Kostas D, *et al.* Dual diagnosis motivational interviewing: a modification of motivational interviewing for substance-abusing patients with psychotic disorders. *Journal of Substance Abuse Treatment.* 2002; **23**: 297–308.

107 Carey KB, Leontieva L, Dimmock J, *et al.* Adapting motivational interventions for comorbid schizophrenia and alcohol use disorders. *Clinical Psychology.* 2007; **14**: 39–57.

108 Harrison TS, Precin P. Cognitive impairments in clients with dual diagnosis: chronic psychotic disorders and substance abuse: considerations for treatment. *Occupational Therapy International.* 1996; **3**: 122–41.

109 Cleaveland BL, Denier CA. Recommendations for health care professionals to improve compliance and treatment outcome among patients with cognitive deficits. *Issues in Mental Health Nursing.* 1998; **19**: 113–24.

110 Carberry H, Burd B. Individual psychotherapy with the brain injured adult. *Cognitive Rehabilitation.* 1986; **5**: 22–4.

111 Evans JJ. Disorders of memory. In: Goldstein LH, McNeil J, editors. *Clinical Neuropsychology: a practical guide to assessment and management.* Chichester: John Wiley & Sons; 2004.

112 Majid MJ, Lincoln NB, Weyman N. Cognitive rehabilitation for memory deficits following stroke. Cochrane Database System Review. 2000; **3**: CD002293.

113 Benedict RH, Shapiro A, Priore R, *et al.* Neuropsychological counseling improves social behavior in cognitively-impaired multiple sclerosis patients. *Multiple Sclerosis.* 2000; **6**: 391–6.

114 Burgess PW, Alderman N, Evans J, *et al.* The ecological validity of tests of executive function. *Journal of the International Neuropsychological Society.* 1998; **4**: 547–58.

115 Addington J, Duchak V. Reasons for substance use in schizophrenia. *Acta Psychiatrica Scandinavica.* 1997; **96**: 329–33.

116 Tiffany ST. A cognitive model of drug urges and drug-use behavior: role of automatic and nonautomatic processes. *Psychology Review.* 1990; **97**: 147–68.

117 Tyerman AD, King NS. *Psychological Approaches to Rehabilitation after Traumatic Brain Injury.* Oxford: Blackwell; 2004.

118 Tyson PJ, Laws KR, Roberts KH, *et al.* Stability of set-shifting and planning abilities in patients with schizophrenia. *Psychiatry Research.* 2004; **129**: 229–39.

119 Spaulding W. Spontaneous and induced changes in cognition during psychiatric rehabilitation. In: Cromwell RL, Snyder CR, editors. *Schizophrenia: innovations in theory and treatment.* New York: Oxford University Press; 1993.

120 Bell M, Bryson G, Wexler BE. Cognitive remediation of working memory deficits: durability of training effects in severely impaired and less severely impaired schizophrenia. *Acta Psychiatrica Scandinavica.* 2003; **108**: 101–9.

121 Medalia A, Revheim N, Casey M. Remediation of problem-solving skills in schizophrenia: evidence of a persistent effect. *Schizophrenia Research.* 2002; **57**: 165–71.

122 Kurtz MM, Moberg PJ, Gur RC, *et al.* Approaches to cognitive remediation of neuropsychological deficits in schizophrenia: a review and meta-analysis. *Neuropsychology Review.* 2001; **11**: 197–210.

123 Twamley EW, Jeste DV, Bellack AS. A review of cognitive training in schizophrenia. *Schizophrenia Bulletin.* 2003; **29**: 359–82.

124 Wykes T, Reeder C, Landau S, *et al.* Cognitive remediation therapy in schizophrenia: randomised controlled trial. *British Journal of Psychiatry.* 2007; **190**: 421–7.

125 Delahunty A, Morice R. *A Training Programme for the Remediation of Cognitive Deficits in Schizophrenia.* Albury, NSW: Department of Health 1993.

126 Wykes T, Reeder C. *Cognitive Remediation Therapy for Schizophrenia.* London: Routledge; 2005.

127 Baddeley A, Wilson BA. When implicit learning fails: amnesia and the problem of error elimination. *Neuropsychologia.* 1994; **32**: 53–68.

128 Wykes T, Reeder C, Williams C, *et al.* Are the effects of cognitive remediation therapy (CRT) durable? Results from an exploratory trial in schizophrenia. *Schizophrenia Research.* 2003; **61**: 163–74.

129 Hayes RL, McGrath JJ. Cognitive rehabilitation for people with schizophrenia and related conditions. *Cochrane Database System Review.* 2000; **3**: CD000968.

130 Sorkin A, Weinshall D, Modai I, *et al.* Improving the accuracy of the diagnosis of schizophrenia by means of virtual reality. *American Journal of Psychiatry.* 2006; **163**: 512–20.

131 Morein-Zamir S, Turner DC, Sahakian BJ. A review of the effects of modafinil on cognition in schizophrenia. *Schizophrenia Bulletin.* 2007; **33**: 1298–306.

132 Sevy S, Rosenthal MH, Alvir J, *et al.* Double-blind, placebo-controlled study of modafinil for fatigue and cognition in schizophrenia patients treated with psychotropic medications. *Journal of Clinical Psychiatry.* 2005; **66**: 839–43.

133 Marx CE, Keefe RS, Buchanan RW, *et al.* Proof-of-concept trial with the neurosteroid pregnenolone targeting cognitive and negative symptoms in schizophrenia. *Neuropsychopharmacology.* 2009; **34**: 1885–903.

134 McGurk SR, Mueser KT, Walling D, *et al.* Cognitive functioning predicts outpatient service utilization in schizophrenia. *Mental Health Service Research.* 2004; **6**: 185–8.

135 Perlick D, Stastny P, Mattis S, *et al.* Contribution of family, cognitive and clinical dimensions to long-term outcome in schizophrenia. *Schizophrenia Research.* 1992; **6**: 257–65.

136 Penk WE, Flannery RB, Jr., Irvin E, *et al.* Characteristics of substance-abusing persons with schizophrenia: the paradox of the dually diagnosed. *Journal of Addictive Diseases.* 2000; **19**: 23–30.

137 McLellan DL. Functional recovery and the principles of disability medicine. In: Wash MS, Oxbury J, editors. *Clinical Neurology.* London: Churchill Livingstone; 1991.

TO LEARN MORE

- Clare L, Wilson BA. *Coping with Memory Problems: a practical guide for people with memory impairments, relatives, friends and careers.* Bury St Edmunds: Thames Valley Test Company; 1997.
- Cleaveland BL, Denier CA. Recommendations for health care professionals to improve compliance and treatment outcome among patients with cognitive deficits. *Issues in Mental Health Nursing.* 1998; **19**: 113–24.
- Goldstein LH, McNeil JE. *Clinical Neuropsychology: a practical guide to assessment and management for clinicians.* Chichester: Wiley; 2004.
- Hodges JR. *Cognitive Assessment for Clinicians.* Oxford: Oxford University Press; 1994.
- Weinstein CS, Shaffer JH. Neurocognitive aspects of substance abuse treatment: a psychotherapist's primer. *Psychotherapy.* 1993; **30**: 317–33.
- Wilson BA, Gracey F, Evans JJ, *et al. Neuropsychological Rehabilitation: theory, models, therapy and outcome.* Cambridge: Cambridge University Press; 2009.

CHAPTER 9

Mental health–substance use first aid

Betty A Kitchener, Anthony F Jorm and Dan I Lubman

PRE-READING EXERCISE 9.1

Time: 10 minutes

Consider the reasons why first aid may be needed for people experiencing mental health–substance use problems. Make notes and review these at the end of this chapter.

THE CONCEPT OF FIRST AID APPLIED TO MENTAL HEALTH AND/OR SUBSTANCE USE PROBLEMS

The concept of 'first aid' is familiar to members of the public in many countries. First aid involves the giving of immediate care to a person who is ill or injured, usually by a lay person who has received some basic training. This first aid is given until more advanced care becomes available or the person's condition improves.

First aid training courses cover physical health crises that may be a threat to life. They generally do not cover mental health or substance use issues with the exception of physical health crises, such as unconsciousness or injury, which may be associated with substance use. Other mental health crises are not covered, such as how to assist a person who is suicidal, self-harming or is acutely psychotic. A more important omission is that first aid courses are typically not oriented to early intervention. They respond to health crises, rather than try to assist people before a crisis develops.

To overcome such omissions, the first aid approaches described in this chapter have been extended to cover both developing mental health and/or substance use problems, as well as crises.[1,2] Here we define Mental Health First Aid as:

> The help offered to a person developing a mental health and/or substance use problem or experiencing a mental health and/or substance use crisis. The first aid is given until appropriate professional help is received or until the crisis resolves.

Mental Health First Aid will typically be offered by someone who is not a mental health or substance use professional, but rather by someone in the person's social network (such as family, friend or work colleague) or someone working in human services (such as a teacher, police officer, employment agency worker).

It is useful to consider where Mental Health First Aid fits into the spectrum of possible interventions for helping people with mental health and/or substance use problems. Figure 9.1 shows the course of a well person who is developing mental health and/or substance use problems. The person may progress to one or more diagnosable disorders, before beginning the process of recovery. There are different types of interventions that may be appropriate at these different stages. If a person is well or has some mild problems, a preventive intervention is appropriate. For a person who is beginning to develop a disorder, an early intervention approach may be more appropriate. For a person who has developed a full-blown disorder, a wide range of clinical treatments may be available to assist the person's recovery. As shown in Figure 9.1, Mental Health First Aid (MHFA) is most appropriate when a person is becoming unwell and is a key approach in facilitating early intervention.

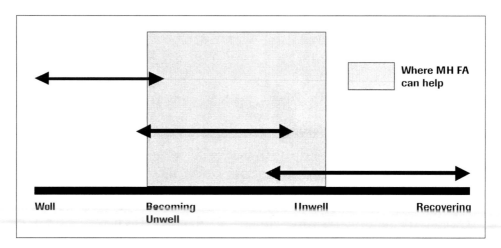

FIGURE 9.1 Spectrum of mental health intervention from wellness to mental disorders and through to recovery, showing the contribution of Mental Health First Aid (MHFA). (Kitchener, Jorm and Kelly;[2] reproduced with permission from the copyright holders.)

WHY FIRST AID IS NEEDED FOR MENTAL HEALTH AND/OR SUBSTANCE USE PROBLEMS

There are many reasons why people who are not mental health or substance use professionals need skills in providing this type of first aid:

➤ **High prevalence of mental health and substance use problems.** National surveys consistently demonstrate high rates of mental health and substance use disorders, including high rates of comorbidity.[3] Such high prevalence rates mean that members of the public will inevitably be interacting with people who have mental health and/or substance use problems.

➤ **Low rates of professional help seeking.** Surveys show low rates of professional help seeking for both mental health and substance use disorders.[4] Even where help is sought there may be delays of many years. This results in people living unnecessarily with the disability associated with mental health and/or substance use problems. It may also mean that their problems become entrenched and thus more difficult to treat. The longer people delay getting professional help the more difficult their recovery can be.[5] In this situation, people close to them can facilitate appropriate help.

➤ **Lack of community knowledge.** Surveys of the public in many countries have shown a lack of knowledge about mental and substance use disorders (e.g. some people cannot recognise these disorders, have negative attitudes towards standard treatments, and are uncertain how to respond to people who have mental health and/or substance use problems).[6] With greater community knowledge about mental health problems, people will be able to recognise these problems in others and be better prepared to offer support.

➤ **Stigmatising attitudes in the community.** Negative attitudes and negative behaviour towards a person with mental health and/or substance use problems may make them less likely to disclose their problems to others, seek professional help and get the social support that can assist their recovery.[7] Better understanding of the experiences of people with mental health and/or substance use problems can reduce prejudice and discrimination.

➤ **Dealing with lack of insight or reluctance to change.** It is not uncommon for people with mental health and/or substance use problems to either be unaware that they have a problem or to be not ready for change. In such situations, those in the person's social network need to know how to respond and provide a supportive relationship, as this is likely to facilitate the person seeking appropriate help over time.

➤ **Professional help is not always available when a mental health and/or substance use problem first arises.** When these sources of help are not available, members of the public can offer immediate first aid and assist the person to get appropriate professional help.

DEVELOPMENT OF MENTAL HEALTH FIRST AID TRAINING

Just as conventional first aid courses are conducted in many countries, Mental Health First Aid courses have been developed to cover developing mental health and substance use problems and associated crisis situations. The world's first Mental Health First Aid training programme began in Australia in 2001,[8,9] in response to a national survey showing poor mental health literacy within the Australian public.[10] The Australian training course involves 12 hours of training. It covers the symptoms, risk factors and first aid strategies for:

➤ depression
➤ anxiety
➤ psychosis
➤ substance misuse.

The course also covers associated crisis situations:

➤ suicidal thoughts and behaviours
➤ non-suicidal self-injury
➤ panic attacks
➤ experiencing a traumatic event
➤ severe psychotic states
➤ acute effects of alcohol use
➤ acute effects of drug use
➤ aggressive behaviours.

The course emphasises the high comorbidity between mental health and substance use problems, and helps first aiders look for mental health problems among people who are misusing substances and to be alert for substance use in people developing mental health problems.

Specialised versions of the Mental Health First Aid training programme have also been developed in Australia. Youth Mental Health First Aid,[11] is designed for adults assisting young people and has additional material on adolescent development, communicating with a young person, and eating disorders. Culturally adapted versions have been produced for Aboriginal and Torres Strait Islander people,[12] and for Australians of Vietnamese background.[13] There is also an e-learning version of the course for people who cannot attend for 12 hours of face-to-face training.[14]

The Mental Health First Aid training course has been evaluated in a number of studies, including three randomised controlled trials and qualitative studies.[8,15–19] These evaluations have shown improvements in knowledge, reduction in stigmatising attitudes, and an increase in help provided to people with mental health or substance use problems.

Because of the need for public skills in this area and the evidence of the Mental Health First Aid programme's effectiveness, it has spread to Canada, Finland, Hong Kong, Japan, New Zealand, Singapore, South Africa, Sweden, Thailand, the UK (with separate programmes in Scotland, England, Wales, Northern Ireland), and the United States. More information is available from the MHFA website: www.mhfa.com.au.

DEVELOPMENT OF GUIDELINES FOR MENTAL HEALTH FIRST AID

With conventional first aid training, there are international guidelines available from the International Liaison Committee on Resuscitation (ILCOR), based on currently available evidence of how to assist in various physical health crisis situations. If Mental Health First Aid training is to also teach evidence-based first aid strategies, similar guidelines are needed about developing mental and substance use disorders and associated crises. However, it is not feasible or ethical to carry out randomised trials of specific Mental Health First Aid strategies (e.g. how a member of the public should assist someone who is suicidal). For this reason, the best available evidence is from a consensus of experts. Accordingly, a series of studies using the Delphi method has recently been carried out to ascertain expert consensus on first aid for a range of mental health and substance use disorders and associated crises.[20–24]

The Delphi method involved recruitment of an international panel of experts rating statements about potential first aid actions that should be included in the guidelines. The panel consisted of three groups:

1   Professionals with expertise in the area.
2   Individuals who have had personal experience of the problem and have reflected on their experiences (e.g. joining advocacy organisations, speaking in public about their experiences or by writing books).
3   Family and caregivers of someone who has had the problem and has been similarly reflective and active.

The first step in each Delphi study was to carry out a systematic review of suggestions made in the literature for first aid actions that are likely to be helpful for that particular disorder or crisis. The literature consisted mainly of lay sources such as websites, and consumer and carer guides. Any first aid suggestion was included, even if it seemed contradictory to other suggestions or was implausible. The aim was to produce a questionnaire that incorporated the full range of potential first aid actions for the expert panels to rate. Rating involved deciding which actions were important to be included in the guidelines. The panel members did not physically meet, but rather provided their views using web-surveys. The results of the survey were fed back to each panel member, giving them the opportunity to revise their opinions or to introduce new ideas not previously considered. Each set of guidelines consisted of first aid actions that 80% or more of each panel agreed should be included.

Guidelines have been produced for how to help someone developing the following disorders:

➤ depression
➤ psychosis
➤ problem drinking
➤ problem drug use
➤ eating disorders.

Guidelines have also been produced for the following crisis situations:

➤ suicidal thoughts and behaviours
➤ non-suicidal self-injury
➤ panic attack
➤ experiencing a traumatic event.

Appropriate first aid actions in these situations may differ from culture to culture and depend on the type of professional services available in a country. For these reasons, work has been carried out to develop consensus first aid guidelines in other cultural groups, such as Australian Aboriginal and Torres Strait Islander people and people in various Asian countries.[25,26] Copies of available guidelines for other cultural groups can be downloaded from: www.mhfa.com.au/Guidelines.shtml.

THE MENTAL HEALTH FIRST AID ACTION PLAN

In any first aid course, participants learn an action plan for the best way to help someone who is injured or ill. A common mnemonic used to remember the procedure for this is DRABC(D), which stands for:

➤ **D**anger
➤ **R**esponse
➤ **A**irway
➤ **B**reathing
➤ **C**irculation
➤ (**D**efibrillation).

Similarly, the Mental Health First Aid programme provides an action plan on how to help a person in a mental health crisis or developing mental health problems. Its mnemonic is ALGEE (*see* Box 9.1).

BOX 9.1 Mental Health First Aid Action Plan

1 **A**pproach the person, assess, and assist with any crisis.
2 **L**isten non-judgementally.
3 **G**ive support and information.
4 **E**ncourage the person to get appropriate professional help.
5 **E**ncourage other supports.

© The Mental Health First Aid Action Plan is reproduced from Kitchener, Jorm and Kelly[2] with permission from the copyright holders.

This action plan contains the major elements found across the set of first aid guidelines developed through expert consensus, referred to above. Each of these actions is explained below:

Action 1: Approach the person, assess and assist with any crisis
The first aider's first task is to approach the person if they think there may be a problem.

The first aider needs to check whether the person is in any crisis and, if so, deal with this. The most likely crises that will be encountered are as follows.
➤ The person may be harming themselves (e.g. attempting suicide, non-suicidal self-injury, alcohol poisoning, overdose).
➤ The person may be experiencing extreme distress (e.g. panic attack, reaction to a traumatic event).
➤ The person's behaviour may be very disturbing to others (e.g. aggression, loss of touch with reality).

The first aider needs to seek professional help immediately if the person appears to be at risk of harming themselves or others, even if the person does not want it.

Assisting with a crisis is the highest priority. However, depending on the situation, the other actions in the Mental Health First Aid Action Plan may need to occur first to facilitate the assessment. The helping person has to use good judgement about the order of these actions and apply them as appropriate.

SELF-ASSESSMENT EXERCISE 9.1

> **Time: 5 minutes**
> **Action 1:** Is there anything you would like to add?

Action 2: Listen non-judgementally

Before being offered specific help for their distress or problem, most people first want to be listened to. Non-judgemental listening involves the listener trying to hear and understand what the other person is saying. This can make it easier for the other person to talk freely about their problems without feeling judged.

SELF-ASSESSMENT EXERCISE 9.2

> **Time: 10 minutes**
> **Action 2:** What qualities will the helper need in order to listen non-judgementally?

Action 3: Give support and information

Once the person has felt listened to, it can be easier to offer them support and information. The support can include emotional support, such as empathising with how the person feels and giving them hope of recovery. It can also include practical help with tasks that may presently seem overwhelming for the person. The first aider can also ask the person if they would like some information and provide it if they do.

SELF-ASSESSMENT EXERCISE 9.3

> **Time: 10 minutes**
> **Action 3:** What actions could be supportive and what might be non-supportive?

Action 4: Encourage the person to get appropriate professional help

People with mental health and/or substance use problems are more likely to recover if they get appropriate professional help. However, they may not know about the options available to them. The person may also need encouragement from the first aider to take the step of seeking professional help.

SELF-ASSESSMENT EXERCISE 9.4

> **Time: 5 minutes**
> **Action 4:** Where might you go in your area to obtain, or find out about, appropriate professional help?

Action 5: Encourage other supports

The first aider can encourage the person to seek the support of family and friends, or of others who have experienced similar problems. There may also be self-help strategies that are helpful for some people.

SELF-ASSESSMENT EXERCISE 9.5

> **Time: 10 minutes**
> *Action 5*: Can you list other types of support that may be helpful?

ILLUSTRATION OF THE ACTION PLAN APPLIED TO A PERSON WITH DEPRESSION AND ALCOHOL PROBLEMS

The first aid responses recommended here are based on the available guidelines (www.mhfa.com.au/Guidelines.shtml), and the Mental Health First Aid training course,[2] and are reproduced here with permission of the copyright holders.

To illustrate the application of the Action Plan, it is applied here to a hypothetical case scenario.

Case study

Dave is a 35-year-old workmate in your organisation. Since his marriage ended six months ago, you and your co-workers have noticed a change in Dave's behaviour and work attendance. He has been taking increasing amounts of sick leave and has been turning up late to work, often smelling strongly of alcohol. He has always been a 'social drinker', regularly meeting up after work on Fridays at the local club. You have noted that Dave has been drinking greater amounts of alcohol over the past six months, as he often remains at the club after everybody else has gone home. Neither you nor your colleagues can recall Dave coming to work smelling of alcohol in the past. Dave is often moody and irritable and is sometimes untidy in appearance when at work. You cannot be sure, but you think he may be depressed. You are concerned about Dave and are worried that his drinking and drop-off in work performance will jeopardise his job. You decide you want to help him by applying the MHFA Action Plan.

SELF-ASSESSMENT EXERCISE 9.6

> **Time: 15 minutes**
> - Make a list of the problems you have identified.
> - What would you need to consider in your initial assessment?

Action 1: Approach the person, assess and assist with any crisis

Approach

Consider the following when making your approach.

➤ **The person's readiness to talk**: Consider Dave's readiness to talk about how he is feeling and his drinking problem by asking about areas of his life that may be affected. For example, his mood, work performance, health and relationships. Is he feeling stressed, distressed or depressed? Let him describe how and why he is feeling this way. Be aware that Dave may deny, or might not recognise, that he has a problem and that trying to force him to admit he has a problem may cause conflict.

➤ **Use 'I' statements**: Express your point of view by using 'I' statements – for example, *'I am concerned about how down you seem and how much you've been drinking lately.'* Identify and discuss Dave's behaviour rather than criticise his character – for example, *'I have noticed that you have been finding it difficult to get to work on time. I know that you are spending more time at the local club after work. I wonder whether your drinking is affecting your mood and is making it difficult for you to get to work in the mornings'*, rather than *'You're a pathetic drunk.'*

➤ **The person's own perception of his drinking**: Try to understand the person's own perception of his drinking. Ask him about his drinking – for example, how much alcohol he tends to drink and if he believes his drinking is a problem.

REFLECTIVE PRACTICE EXERCISE 9.1

> **Time: 15 minutes**
> Plan how you will approach Dave about your concerns regarding his drinking and possible depressed mood.

Choose a suitable time when both you and Dave are available to talk where there will be no interruptions, as well as a space where you both feel comfortable and when both of you are sober and in a calm frame of mind. Tell Dave that you are concerned about how he is feeling and how much he is drinking lately. Say that you have noticed he is not working so well and has been off sick a fair bit. Ask him how things have been going for him.

At first, Dave may tell you that nothing is wrong and not to worry about him – he has simply been feeling off-colour. He may admit that he has been drinking a little bit more lately, but that you should not be concerned as he will cut back his drinking when he feels better.

Assess

There are six main crises that may be associated with depressed mood and problem drinking:

1 The person is **intoxicated**
2 The person has **alcohol poisoning**

3 The person is in **severe withdrawal**
4 The person is **aggressive**
5 The person has **suicidal thoughts and/or behaviours**
6 The person is engaging in **non-suicidal self-injury**.

The first four crises (**intoxication, alcohol poisoning, severe withdrawal** and **aggression**) will be observed more in the behaviour of the person than what they tell you, whereas the last two crises (**suicidal thoughts and for behaviours** and **non-suicidal self-injury**) may only become apparent after you have approached the person about your concerns.

KEY POINT 9.1

A person who is depressed and also has an alcohol problem has a much higher risk of suicide and self-injury.

If you have concerns that the person is in crisis, move on to Assist. If you have no concerns that the person is in crisis, move on to Action 2.

Given Dave's reply and what you have observed, you will need to assess him more fully, as you suspect that he is really not doing well. You tell him that you are really worried about him, as you know that when people drink heavily and get down, they can think that life is not worth living. You say to him, '*I am concerned that you might have been thinking about suicide.*'

Dave reacts to your question with: '*Don't worry – I wouldn't kill myself – I'm just a bit down, the drink is just to take the edge off it. I can handle my drinking – I don't have a problem – Don't worry about me.*' With Dave reacting like this, you believe there is no current crisis to assist with. You confirm that you just want to make sure he is alright and that you are there to help him. You move on to Action 2.

SELF ASSESSMENT EXERCISE 9.7

Time: 10 minutes
What skills would you need in order to act supportively at this stage?

Action 2: Listen non-judgementally

Listening non-judgementally is important at this stage as it can help Dave to feel heard and understood, while not being judged in any way. If you believe Dave is not in a crisis that needs immediate attention, you can engage him in conversation, such as asking him about how he is feeling and how long he has been feeling this way. This may help him feel more comfortable to talk freely about his problems and to ask for help. This conversation might be the first time he has thought about his drinking as a problem. Important actions include:

➤ listening without judging Dave as bad or immoral
➤ avoiding expressing moral judgements about his drinking

➤ not being critical of Dave; you are more likely to be able to help him over the long term if you maintain a non-critical but concerned approach

➤ not labelling him (e.g. an 'addict') or accusing him of being an alcoholic

➤ not expressing your frustration at him for having alcohol problems.

Tips for non-judgemental listening

It is very difficult to be entirely non-judgemental all of the time. We automatically make judgements about people from the minute we first see or meet them, based on their appearance, behaviour and what they say. In spite of any emotional response you have, you need to continue listening respectfully and avoid expressing a negative reaction to what the person says. This is sometimes difficult, and may be made more complex by your relationship with the person or your personal beliefs about their situation. You need to set aside these beliefs and reactions in order to focus on the needs of the person you are helping: to be heard, understood and helped. Remember that you are providing the person with a safe space to express themselves, and a negative reaction from you can prevent them from feeling that sense of safety.

You can be an effective non-judgemental listener by paying special attention to two main areas:

➤ your **attitudes**, and how they are conveyed, and

➤ effective **communication skills** – both verbal and non-verbal.

SELF-ASSESSMENT EXERCISE 9.8

Time: 15 minutes

Consider your own non-verbal communication. What cues can you give to demonstrate you are listening?

The **key attitudes** involved in non-judgemental listening are acceptance, genuineness and empathy. Using the following simple **verbal skills** will show that you are listening.

➤ Ask questions which show that you genuinely care and want clarification about what the person is saying.

➤ Check your understanding by restating what they have said and summarising facts and feelings.

➤ Listen not only to what the person says but how they say it; their tone of voice and non-verbal cues will give extra clues about how they are feeling.

➤ Use minimal prompts, such as 'I see' and 'Ah' when necessary to keep the conversation going.

➤ Be patient, even when the person may not be communicating well, may be repetitive or may be speaking slower and less clearly than usual.

➤ Do not be critical of them and do not express your frustration at the person for having such problems.

➤ Avoid giving unhelpful advice such as 'pull yourself together' or 'cheer up'. If this was possible the person would do it.

➤ Do not interrupt the person when they are speaking, especially to share your opinions or experiences.
➤ Avoid confrontation unless necessary to prevent harmful or dangerous acts.
➤ Remember that pauses and silences are okay.

Keep the following **non-verbal cues** in mind to reinforce your non-judgemental listening:
➤ Pay close attention to what the person says.
➤ Maintain comfortable eye contact. Do not avoid eye contact, but do avoid staring; you can do this by maintaining the level of eye contact that the person seems most comfortable with.
➤ Maintain an open body position. Don't cross your arms over your body, as this may appear defensive.
➤ Sit down, even if the person is standing, as this seems less threatening.
➤ It is best to sit alongside the person and angled towards them, rather than directly opposite them.
➤ Do not fidget.

You assure Dave that you just want to make sure he is all right and that you are there to help him – not to judge him. You ask Dave how long he has been feeling down. You follow up with questions about anything in his life that may have led to this. You listen to Dave talk about his low mood and his marriage breakdown without judging him. You do not make any negative comments about his drinking. You are not critical of him because you know that you are more likely to be able to help Dave in the long term if you maintain a non-critical approach.

As you continue to listen to him, Dave begins to open up more. He lets you know that he recently had a drink-driving charge and that he has been suffering with other health problems including a stomach ulcer, which is why he has been off sick more than usual. He also tells you that his private life has been very difficult over the past year.

Dave sits down and holds his head low. He wipes his eyes with his hands. He tells you that he cannot seem to stop drinking – that as soon as he feels down or stressed, the first thing he does is look for a drink. He just cannot seem to control himself. He does not know what to do or who to turn to. He feels embarrassed that he has got this way.

Action 3: Give support and information
Try to incorporate the following considerations.
➤ Treat Dave with respect and dignity. Each person's situation and needs are unique.
➤ Do not blame him for his problems. Depression and alcohol misuse are real health issues. It is important to remind him that he has a health problem and that he is not to blame for feeling 'down'.
➤ Have realistic expectations for Dave. Let him know that he is not weak or a failure because he has these health problems, and that you do not think less of

him as a person. You should acknowledge that he is not 'faking', 'lazy', 'weak' or 'selfish'.

➤ Offer consistent emotional support and understanding. It is more important for you to be genuinely caring than for you to say all the 'right things'. It is important to be patient, persistent and encouraging when supporting someone with depression and alcohol problems. You should also offer him kindness and attention, even if it is not reciprocated. Aim to be consistent and predictable in your interactions with Dave.

➤ Give him hope for recovery. You need to encourage Dave that, with time and treatment, he will feel better. Offer emotional support and hope of a more positive future in whatever form he will accept.

➤ Provide practical help. Ask Dave if he would like any practical assistance with tasks but be careful not to take over or encourage dependency.

➤ Offer information. Ask Dave if he would like some information about depression and alcohol. If he does want some information, it is important that you give him resources that are accurate and appropriate to his situation.

➤ Do not expect a change in Dave's thinking or behaviour right away. Major behaviour changes take time to achieve and often involve a person going through a number of stages. Bear in mind that:
— changing drinking habits is not easy
— a person's willpower and self-resolve is not always enough to help them stop problem drinking or to change a depressed mood
— giving advice alone may not help the person change their mood and behaviour.

You tell Dave that you understand he has had a rough time and that the way he is handling it is very common. You tell him that he has taken a huge step in acknowledging that he has a problem.

It is important to convey to Dave that things can be better. You tell him that drinking problems are common and that there are programmes available to help people deal with alcohol and mood problems.

Dave agrees that his drinking has increased, but says he is finding it difficult to do something about it at the moment as the alcohol helps him to cope. You ask him if he would like some information about depression and about drinking at a low-risk level. Dave agrees that could be a good idea and you give him some pamphlets. The alcohol pamphlet contains the information in Box 9.2:

BOX 9.2 Practical tips for low-risk drinking

- Know what a standard drink is and the number of standard drinks you consume.
- Switch to non-alcoholic drinks when you start to feel the effects of alcohol.
- Do not let people top up your drink before it is finished, so as not to lose track of how much alcohol you have consumed.
- Avoid keeping up with your friends drink for drink.
- Avoid drinking competitions and drinking games.

- Drink slowly; for example, by taking sips instead of gulps and putting your drink down between sips.
- Have one drink at a time.
- Spend your time in activities that don't involve drinking.
- Make drinking alcohol a complementary activity instead of the sole activity.
- Identify situations where drinking is likely and avoid them if practical.

Action 4: Encourage the person to get appropriate professional help

Professional help is warranted when depression lasts for weeks and affects a person's functioning in daily life. People with depressive disorders are more likely to seek help if someone close to them suggests it.[27]

Ask Dave if he needs help to manage how he is feeling. If he feels he does need help, discuss the options that he has for seeking help and encourage him to use these options. If Dave does not know where to get help, offer to help him seek assistance. It is important to encourage him to get appropriate professional help and effective treatment as early as possible.

A variety of health professionals can provide help to a person with depression and alcohol problems. They are:

➤ general practitioners
➤ psychologists
➤ drug and alcohol specialists
➤ psychiatrists.

Most people recover from depression and alcohol problems and lead satisfying and productive lives. There are a range of treatments that are effective in the treatment of depression and also alcohol problems.

Treatments for depression and problem alcohol use depend on the severity of the problem, how motivated the person is to change, and what other physical and mental health problems they also have.

If Dave has a mood and an alcohol use disorder, treatment needs to help him to:

➤ learn skills to overcome depression
➤ overcome any physiological dependence on alcohol (e.g. managing withdrawals)
➤ overcome any psychological dependence (e.g. coping with cravings, not being able to control his level of drinking)
➤ overcome any habits around drinking that have been formed (e.g. a social life that revolves around drinking).

SELF-ASSESSMENT EXERCISE 9.9

Time: 10 minutes
Make a list of, and reflect on, the possible reasons why Dave may not want help.

What if the person doesn't want help?

Dave may not want professional help when it is first suggested to him and may find it difficult to accept. You should find out if there are specific reasons why this is the case. For example, he might be concerned about the cost of treatment, or about not having a health professional he likes, or being told to stop drinking alcohol completely, or he might be worried he will be sent to hospital. These reasons may be based on mistaken beliefs and, if so, you may be able to help him overcome any worries he has about seeking help. Reassure Dave that professional help is confidential.

If Dave still does not want help after you have explored this with him, let him know that if he changes his mind in the future about seeking help he can contact you. You must respect Dave's right not to seek help unless you believe that he is at risk of harming himself or others. However, if his drinking is causing problems, you should set boundaries around what behaviour you are willing and not willing to accept from him. Be prepared to talk to Dave about seeking professional help again in the future. Be compassionate and patient while waiting for Dave to accept he needs professional help – it is ultimately his decision.

You suggest to Dave that it might be wise for him to see a professional to help him through his problems. Dave does not seem keen about talking to anyone else about his problems. When you ask him why, he replies that doctors just give you pills and he does not want to take any pills because he then will not be able to drink alcohol. You tell him that there are other alternatives to taking medication and he could see a counsellor, such as a mental health professional, a drug and alcohol professional or the Employee Assistance Programme at his workplace. You tell Dave that your brother-in-law used the Employee Assistance Programme at his workplace and found it really useful. No one at his work knew that he was getting this counselling.

Dave agrees he needs to see someone, but says he is not ready to talk to anyone about his problems. You realise that if Dave is to get help eventually, you need to keep a good relationship with him and continue to be supportive. You do not make any critical comments on the fact that he does not want to seek help right now. You tell him that it is his decision to make and you are happy to keep talking with him in the future if he finds that helpful.

SELF-ASSESSMENT EXERCISE 9.10

> **Time: 20 minutes**
> - What measures do you think a family could take in order to provide support at home?
> - How might the family be supported?

Action 5: Encourage other supports

Encourage Dave to consider other supports available to him, such as family, friends, and support group, and self-help strategies. Recovery is quicker for people who feel supported by those around them. Research has shown that people with substance use problems are more likely to recover if:[28]

➤ they have stable family relationships

> ➤ they are not treated with criticism and hostility by their family
> ➤ they have supportive friends
> ➤ their friends do not use alcohol or drugs themselves and they encourage the person not to use.

Family and friends can also play an important role in the recovery of a person with depression.[29] Encourage Dave to reach out to friends and family who support his efforts to change his drinking behaviours and to spend time with supportive non-drinking friends and family. Family and friends can help Dave to seek treatment and support a change in his drinking. They can also help reduce the chances of a relapse after he has stopped drinking. People are more likely to start using again if there is an emotional upset in their life; family and friends can try to reduce this possibility. It may be appropriate to warn Dave that not all family and friends will be supportive of his efforts to cut down his drinking.

Some people who experience depression and alcohol problems find it helpful to meet with other people who have had similar experiences. There are numerous groups that support individuals who are recovering from substance use by providing mutual support and information, including Alcoholics Anonymous (AA) and Narcotics Anonymous (NA). Research shows that these groups can be beneficial.[30]

You ask if there is anyone in his family or friends who he could speak to about his problems. Dave says that his mother has always been a supportive person, but he does not get on well with his father. You discuss with Dave whether his mother could be someone he could talk to. You also suggest the possibility of going to a support group. You tell him about the alcohol support group a friend of yours has attended. Dave says he might think about this and you offer to get him the contact number of the group.

Because you want to keep communication going with Dave, you propose that you meet for lunch once a week. This will give you the opportunity to be a supportive listener for Dave and facilitate professional help seeking when he is ready for it.

CONCLUSION

Mental health–substance use problems are highly prevalent in our community. However, there is considerable stigma surrounding these disorders, and professional help seeking is generally low. If we are to reduce the individual and community costs associated with these disorders, it is imperative that we are all better informed and trained in providing help to a person developing a mental health and/or substance use problem or experiencing a mental health and/or substance use crisis. Mental Health First Aid is an internationally applicable training programme that has been shown to be acceptable and effective. The course is based on international consensus-based guidelines that have been developed to cover a broad range of mental health and substance use problems. We suggest that such an early intervention approach is likely to assist in the destigmatising of mental health and substance use problems and substantially reduce the delay in professional help seeking for these disorders.

REFERENCES

1 Kitchener BA, Jorm AF. *Mental Health First Aid Manual.* Canberra, ACT: Centre for Mental Health Research; 2002.

2 Kitchener BA, Jorm AF, Kelly CM. *Mental Health First Aid Manual. Second edition.* Melbourne, VIC: Orygen Youth Health Research Centre; 2010.

3 Kessler RC, Angermeyer M, Anthony JC, *et al.* Lifetime prevalence and age-of-onset distributions of mental disorders in the World Health Organization's World Mental Health Survey Initiative. *World Psychiatry.* 2007; **6**: 168–76.

4 Wang PS, Angermeyer M, Borges G, *et al.* Delay and failure in treatment seeking after first onset of mental disorders in the World Health Organization's World Mental Health Survey Initiative. *World Psychiatry.* 2007; **6**: 177–85.

5 Marshall M, Lewis S, Lockwood A, *et al.* Association between duration of untreated psychosis and outcome in cohorts of first-episode patients: a systematic review. *Archives of General Psychiatry.* 2005; **62**: 975–83.

6 Jorm AF, Kelly CM. Improving the public's understanding and response to mental disorders. *Australian Psychologist.* 2007; **42**: 81–9.

7 Schomerus G, Angermeyer MC. Stigma and its impact on help-seeking for mental disorders: what do we know? *Epidemiologiae psichiatria sociale.* 2008; **17**: 1–9.

8 Kitchener BA, Jorm AF. Mental health first aid training for the public: evaluation of effects on knowledge, attitudes and helping behavior. *BMC Psychiatry.* 2002; **2**: 10.

9 Kitchener BA, Jorm AF. Mental health first aid: an international programme for early intervention. *Early Intervention in Psychiatry.* 2008; **2**: 55–61.

10 Jorm AF, Korten AE, Jacomb PA, *et al.* 'Mental health literacy': a survey of the public's ability to recognise mental disorders and their beliefs about the effectiveness of treatment. *Medical Journal of Australia.* 1997; **166**: 182–6.

11 Kitchener BA, Jorm AF. *Youth Mental Health First Aid: a manual for adults assisting youth.* Melbourne, VIC: Orygen Research Centre; 2007.

12 Kanowski LG, Kitchener BA, Jorm AF, editors. *Aboriginal and Torres Strait Islander Mental Health First Aid Manual.* Melbourne, VIC: Orygen Research Centre; 2008.

13 Kitchener BA, Jorm AF, Kanowski LG. *Cam Nang Cap Cuu Tam Than: Vietnamese Mental Health First Aid Manual.* Melbourne, VIC: Orygen Research Centre, 2008.

14 Kitchener BA, Jorm AF. *Mental Health First Aid: an e-learning course.* Melbourne, VIC: Orygen Research Centre; 2008.

15 Jorm AF, Kitchener BA, O'Kearney R, *et al.* Mental health first aid training of the public in a rural area: a cluster randomized trial [ISRCTN53887541]. *BMC Psychiatry.* 2004; **4**: 33.

16 Kitchener BA, Jorm AF. Mental health first aid training in a workplace setting: a randomized controlled trial [ISRCTN13249129]. *BMC Psychiatry.* 2004; **4**: 23.

17 Jorm AF, Kitchener BA, Mugford SK. Experiences in applying skills learned in a mental health first aid training course: a qualitative study of participants' stories. *BMC Psychiatry.* 2005; **5**: 43.

18 Sartore GM, Kelly B, Stain HJ, *et al.* Improving mental health capacity in rural communities: mental health first aid delivery in drought-affected rural New South Wales. *Australian Journal of Rural Health.* 2008; **16**: 313–18.

19 Jorm AF, Kitchener BA, Sawyer MG, *et al.* Mental health first aid training for high school teachers: a cluster randomized trial. *BMC Psychiatry.* 2010; **10**: 51.

20 Kelly CM, Jorm AF, Kitchener BA, *et al.* Development of mental health first aid guidelines for non-suicidal self-injury: a Delphi study. *BMC Psychiatry.* 2008; **8**: 62.

21 Kelly CM, Jorm AF, Kitchener BA, *et al.* Development of mental health first aid guidelines for suicidal ideation and behaviour: a Delphi study. *BMC Psychiatry.* 2008; **8**: 17.

22 Langlands RL, Jorm AF, Kelly, CM, *et al.* First aid recommendations for psychosis: using the Delphi method to gain consensus between mental health consumers, carers and clinicians. *Schizophrenia Bulletin.* 2008; **34**: 435–43.

23 Langlands RL, Jorm, AF, Kelly CM, *et al.* First aid for depression: a Delphi consensus study with consumers, carers and clinicians. *Journal of Affective Disorders.* 2008; **105**: 157–65.

24 Kingston AH, Jorm AF, Kitchener BA, *et al.* Helping someone with problem drinking: mental health first aid guidelines – a Delphi expert consensus study. *BMC Psychiatry.* 2009; **9**: 79.

25 Hart LM, Jorm AF, Kanowski LG, *et al.* Mental health first aid for Indigenous Australians: using Delphi consensus studies to develop guidelines for culturally appropriate responses to mental health problems. *BMC Psychiatry.* 2009; **9**: 47.

26 Jorm AF, Minas H, Langlands RL, *et al.* First aid guidelines for psychosis in Asian countries: a Delphi consensus study. *International Journal of Mental Health Systems.* 2008; **2**: 2.

27 Dew MA, Bromet EJ, Schulberg HC, *et al.* Factors affecting service utilization for depression in a white collar population. *Social Psychiatry and Psychiatric Epidemiology.* 1991; **26**: 230–7.

28 Moos RH. Theory-based processes that promote the remission of substance use disorders. *Clinical Psychology Review.* 2007; **27**: 537–51.

29 Keitner GI, Ryan CE, Miller IW, *et al.* Role of the family in recovery and major depression. *American Journal of Psychiatry.* 1995; **152**: 1002–8.

30 Kelly JF. Self-help for substance-use disorders: history, effectiveness, knowledge gaps, and research opportunities. *Clinical Psychology Review.* 2003; **23**: 639–63.

TO LEARN MORE

- Mental Health First Aid Guidelines: www.mhfa.com.au/Guidelines.shtml
- e-learning Mental Health First Aid: www.mhfa.com.au/elearning_mhfa.shtml

Mental health–substance use: why do general practitioners need to know about it?

Chris Holmwood

WHAT IS DIFFERENT ABOUT GENERAL PRACTICE AND ITS APPROACHES TO COMORBIDITY?

Barbara Starfield[1] defines the essential elements of general practice and primary care as:

- **accessibility of services** in terms of hours open, booking availability, and the services themselves being physically accessible
- **the range of services** available enable the person to gain assistance with a broad range of problems with virtually no exceptions
- **a defined population served** by the service enables a primary care system to address health problems from a population health perspective
- **continuity** that enables a person to receive care across a long period of time.

The primary care clinician therefore can approach the person experiencing comorbid mental health–substance use problems in a manner that is subtly different from the approaches of other services.

PATTERNS OF MENTAL HEALTH–SUBSTANCE USE AND CONCEPTUAL ISSUES RELEVANT TO GENERAL PRACTICE

General practice and other primary care services experience a range of competing priorities all jostling for the clinician's attention. The very breadth of practice (i.e. *range of services*) undertaken in these settings, while one of its strengths, also presents great difficulties. Mental health and substance use-related problems are just one (albeit common) group of problems that the clinician may encounter in the primary care setting.

Mental health–substance use patterns vary depending on the populations under study. The two most important populations to consider from a primary care perspective are the general community and the sub-group who actually seek help from their general practitioner or primary health service. Population-based studies (such

119

as the Epidemiological Catchment Area Study[2] [US] or the National Comorbidity Survey[3] [US]), look at the prevalence of mental disorders and substance use disorders of people in the community, most of whom will not seek help for their problem.

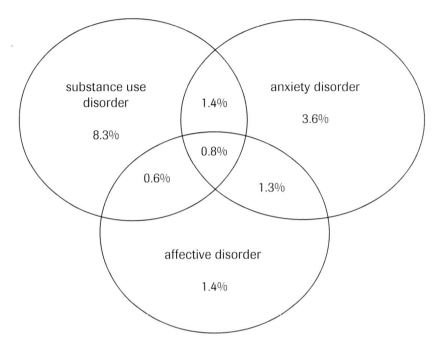

FIGURE 10.1 Patterns of mental health–substance use (Patterns of comorbidity in the male Australian Community, *National Survey of Mental Health and Wellbeing*, 1997 [Australia][6])

However, most people with a psychological problem will not seek assistance for this. In the 2007 Australian National Survey of Mental Health and Wellbeing[4] only 35% of people experiencing mental health–substance use disorders actually accessed any service for assistance. It follows that patterns will be different among those who actually present to a health service. Moreover, patterns of mental health–substance use seen in general practice will be different from those seen in specialty mental health or substance use services.

Even within primary care or general practice, patterns will vary depending on the *populations being served* (e.g. prisons, refugee communities, younger populations in new housing developments, etc.).

Within general practice mental health–substance use disorders are common and related to cumulative increases in disability.[5] The common comorbidities in general practice involve alcohol and the high prevalence mental disorders, such as depression and the anxiety disorders. Of course the patterns of problematic substance use will vary from one country to another, depending on different background rates of the use of different substances.

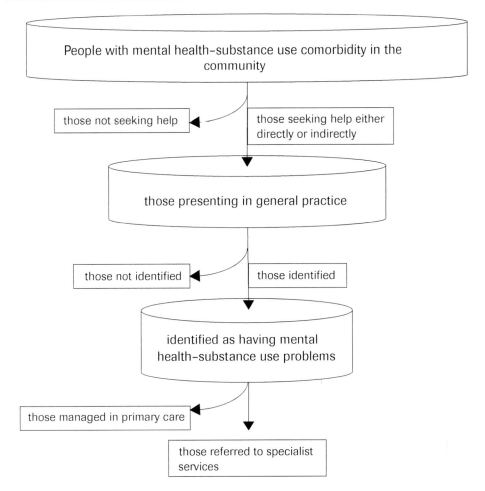

FIGURE 10.2 Prevalence and detection of mental health–substance use in the community, primary care and specialist settings[6]

Figure 10.2 demonstrates how different service-related 'sieves' end up determining different groups with different characteristics. For example, community samples will be different from primary care samples, which will in turn be different from those who are diagnosed and treated or referred to more specialised services.

Conceptually, mental health–substance use does not present difficulties for general practitioners (GPs) because they are very much used to caring for people with multiple problems running in parallel. In contrast, specialist mental health or substance use services can run into difficulty with mental health–substance use because of arbitrary demarcation regarding what types of clinical problems they manage, lack of clarity about the aetiology of the person's problem, and the best way to manage them (e.g. methamphetamine or cannabis-induced or exacerbated psychotic disorders).

However, mental health–substance use can present particular problems for GPs because people experience increased levels of disability, and identification and management of one problem is hampered by the other.

In addition, the conundrum of what constitutes 'caseness' or an actual disorder in general practice continues to be debated. Most instruments used for screening, or for population-based surveys, look at mental disorder or substance use-related problems as dimensional. At some point along the dimension people are categorised as having a 'disorder'. So what we have is a set of diagnostic tools that are in fact dimensional but seduce us into thinking categorically (does the person have a disorder or not?). This set point can vary depending on the purpose for which the instrument is used.

In the general practice setting we often face people with sub-threshold complexes of symptoms of depression and anxiety, as well as non-dependent but nevertheless harmful levels of substance use, all rolled into one. Whether they actually have a diagnosable 'disorder' is somewhat academic if they present as distressed. Primary care services do not have the privilege of judging a person 'not for service'.

DETECTION

Especially within the general practice or primary care setting, mental disorders and substance use disorders are frequently not identified or not addressed.[7-8] Given that in the community setting people will frequently present with somatic symptoms, it is hardly surprising that psychological problems go unidentified.

In addition, despite substance use being quite common in most communities, rates of questioning and recording information of the individuals' tobacco and alcohol use remains low.[9] It is a case of not knowing if you are not asking. In the case of alcohol, for instance, most morbidity associated with alcohol use is by people who are not dependent drinkers so that there will frequently be no clues to their drinking patterns despite them being hazardous.[10]

KEY POINT 10.1

Given that detection of mental health or substance use-related problems are not optimal in the general practice setting, if either *is* identified, the other should automatically be sought, e.g. whenever they become aware that the individual may have a mental health problem, they should also enquire about substance use.

Case study 10.1 Part I

Peter is a 19-year-old man who has attended your general practice in a regional centre a few times over the past five years with occasional intercurrent illnesses and minor sports-related injuries. You see him one morning for the removal of sutures from a scalp laceration that he sustained after a fall outside a bar the week before. He's had a tetanus shot and feels fine. The wound is well healed.

SELF-ASSESSMENT EXERCISE 10.1

> **Time: 10 minutes**
> What issues might you want to explore with Peter?

We know that substance use is common in this age group. The fact that Paul sustained an injury and that it occurred near premises licensed to supply alcohol would make further exploration of alcohol use a logical next step. Some open-ended questions about Paul's life functioning, family and social situation and then alcohol use might give the GP a much better idea of the context of the injury.

Case study 10.1 Part II

Peter can't actually remember how much he drank that night. However, in general when he goes out to socialise he has about 100–150 g of alcohol as spirits and beer. He only drinks when he socialises, which is generally on weekends and not during the week. Two years ago he was convicted of a drink-driving offence.

SELF-ASSESSMENT EXERCISE 10.2

> **Time: 5 minutes**
> What other information might you want from Peter?

The next step might be to try to better determine the pattern of alcohol use, Peter's feelings about his alcohol use and the reasons why he does drink. This information will help determine the level of risk and whether he is alcohol dependent. In addition, it will assist with a brief intervention (*see* Book 4, Chapter 8) or motivational interviewing (*see* Book 4, Chapter 7).[11] Finally, this might give the GP some clues about whether Peter might be experiencing an underlying mental disorder that is triggering his drinking, or being made worse by his drinking.

Case study 10.1 Part III

It turns out that Peter drinks to settle his nerves when he is socialising. He says that he does get very anxious when socialising and he has found that alcohol settles this anxiety. Over the past four years he has depended on the alcohol during these sorts of activities, but he does not experience withdrawal symptoms and apart from when he socialises he does not feel any compulsion to drink.

SELF-ASSESSMENT EXERCISE 10.3

> **Time: 10 minutes**
> What might you observe/look for here? What questions might you ask?

So, in Peter's situation, his initial presentation for removal of sutures is relatively innocuous. Through some opportunistic questioning it turns out that Peter's alcohol use presents at least a moderate risk. It also emerges (following that the clinician should look for mental health problems in people presenting like Peter) that he has an underlying social phobia.

One of the unique things about primary care and general practice is that people present for a range of problems, some of which may be related to mental health problems, some of which are related to substance use, or both. Most of these people will never present to specialist mental health services or to substance use services. However, they are the group that experiences the greatest burden of disability when considered across the population.[12]

Looking at detection of psychological distress in general, we might know that listening skill such as the following increase detection of psychological problems:[13]

➤ using eye contact
➤ using directive 'open' questions rather than closed questions initially
➤ question 'coning', leaving closed questions to the end to clarify uncertainties
➤ making sure the GP clarifies what the individual originally has come for.

These skills can be learnt relatively easily using video recordings of interviews and feedback.[14,15]

If a mental health problem has been identified, it is then a small step to enquire about a person's alcohol or other substance use as a matter of course. It is important to try to develop an understanding of the relationship between the person's substance use, their mental health problems, their general health and general life stressors.

Other triggers for suspecting that comorbidity might be an underlying issue are:[16]

➤ when the GP is treating one disorder and progress is slower than expected
➤ when there are problems with non-attendance for appointments
➤ when the individual presents frequently
➤ when there are requests for analgesics or benzodiazepines
➤ when the presenting physical problems are vague and difficult to diagnose
➤ when there has been trauma related to intoxication
➤ when there is a family history of substance use-related problems or mental disorder.

ASSESSMENT

General practice has some unique characteristics that make approaches to assessment quite different from the way specialist services might assess mental health–substance use.

Length of consultation varies from country to country, but primary care consultations are on average relatively short (7–15 minutes).[17,18] Even within countries there is considerable variation of length of consultation. Therefore, the GP when faced with a complex set of problems will deal with them by having some longer consultations, or dealing with the problems through a series of standard length consultations. Care tends to be episodic and each episode brief.

Another defining feature of general practice is *continuity of care* for the individual over several years. What general practice and primary care miss out on in terms of duration of consultation, they benefit from in terms of frequency of consultation and this capacity to provide care over an often extended period of time. In the case of mental health–substance use disorder, this continuity of care allows an opportunistic approach to helping the individual that may not be possible in other settings.

Case study 10.2 Part I

Maria has paranoid schizophrenia and receives her depo-antipsychotic from her general practice on a fortnightly basis through the mental health outreach nurse. She smokes cannabis on a daily basis. Maria has about five cones per day that she smokes using a water pipe. She mixes it 50/50 with tobacco. She is on a disability support pension. Her positive symptoms are under control and do not worry her that much, but she lacks energy and motivation and has a chronically depressed mood. She does not see that her cannabis use is a problem.

SELF-ASSESSMENT EXERCISE 10.4

Time: 10 minutes
What might the approach be here?

Maria has some significant negative symptoms. These may be due to her schizophrenia, to the cannabis, or she may have a concurrent depressive disorder. From stages of change perspective[19] (*see* Book 4, Chapter 6), she is a pre-contemplator regarding her cannabis use. Despite some probing on several occasions, Maria is resistant to cutting down her cannabis use. She feels that it reduced her boredom and lifts her mood.

Case study 10.2 Part II

One winter Maria develops a pneumonia requiring hospital admission and is quite ill for several weeks after discharge. You are seeing her for some persistent dyspnoea on exertion and cough. These are gradually resolving but progress is slow. Maria brings up her cannabis and tobacco use and wonders whether they may be making her chest problems slow to resolve.

SELF-ASSESSMENT EXERCISE 10.5

Time: 10 minutes
How would you respond?

Something has changed here with Maria. Her readiness for change with her cannabis use has moved from the pre-contemplation stage to the contemplation stage, as a result of a physical health problem. This scenario demonstrates that general practice offers some opportunities over time to help people with their mental health–substance use problems that might not have been possible if she had been attending a specialist service. The presentation because of the pneumonia and its sequelae, the link with the cannabis use, the possible links between the cannabis and the negative symptoms, all align to allow the GP to help her with a significant change that will probably improve both her general health and her mental health. How the GP might respond will be dealt with in the next section.

Assessment needs to include the following.

➤ What are the patterns of use of the substance? What is the risk associated with the use? Is the use dependent? What harms are already occurring?

➤ What are the positive outcomes that the individual experiences about their substance use?

➤ What are the psychological symptoms?

➤ How disabled is the person? What is the effect of their problems on their functioning at home, work, study, socially, and so on?

➤ (How) do the mental health problems and the substance use relate to one another?

➤ Most important, what does the individual think about all of the above? Do they want to change? How might they change?

The GP can address these issues over multiple contacts sometimes over an extensive period of time. The GP's response can be opportunistic. If the individual is resistant to change, the GP can at least help with aspects of their physical health. When the opportunity arises, when there is a 'chink in the armour' of resistance, a glimmer of insight or doubt, the GP can take advantage of this to help the individual move towards some change.

KEY POINT 10.2

The assessment of individuals should be flexible and not be particularly bound by diagnostic categories. The great proportion of burden of illness on a population basis occurs in people with mixed symptomatology.

INTERVENTIONS

There are no real 'mental health–substance use-specific' interventions. The skills needed are a combination of those needed for helping people with substance use-related problems; with those needed for mental health problems, *as well as* an understanding of the interplay between substance use and mental health and when to apply the different types of interventions.

General practice and primary care are constantly evolving in many countries. General practices per se are becoming much more multidisciplinary in the nature of the work they do and the services they provide. It is not uncommon now for general practices to have community psychiatric nurses, primary care counsellors, clinical psychologists and sometimes visiting psychiatrists all providing a range of services from the one site, as well as the general practitioners themselves. The following range of interventions does not apply to any one particular professional, but rather to the general practice or primary care service itself, involving some or all of the different clinicians working in that setting.

Determining and responding to different levels of readiness for change

One of the key things to consider when sorting out *what to do* is to determine the individual's readiness for change or insight. The individual's insight or readiness for change will vary over time and may be different for their mental health problem and their substance use.

The 'trans-theoretical model'[19] looks at stages of readiness for change (*see* Figure 10.3 and *see also* Book 4, Chapter 6). The stages of change often used are as follows.

➤ **Precontemplation**: the non-reflective person not yet thinking about their behaviour as problematic.
➤ **Contemplation**: starting to think about their substance use.
➤ **Preparation**: making active preparatory steps towards changing.
➤ **Action**: actually putting the plans into action.

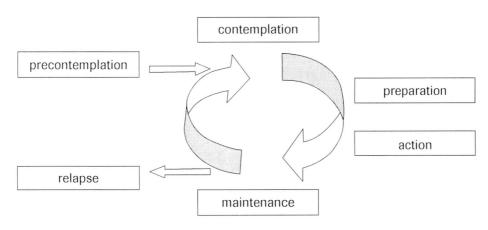

FIGURE 10.3 Stages of change model

➤ **Maintenance**: developing and acting out a range of strategies for maintaining the changed behaviour.
➤ **Relapse**: recognising that some behaviour will be chronic and difficult to change permanently.

The value of general practice lies in the continuity of care it provides, the development of long-term therapeutic relationships and the capacity of the GP to intervene opportunistically.

Information giving

Because there will be episodic but regular contact with the individual over time, there will be opportunities for giving individuals information about their mental health problem or their substance use, even if they are not ready for change.

Individuals respect their general practitioners as sources of unbiased information about their health, including alcohol,[20] and if the message is *'This is just for your information. I respect your right to decide what is best for you'* it will be well received – even if it does not elicit any immediate change in behaviour! Of course some judgement needs to be used regarding the person's receptiveness to such information. In any clinical setting maintenance of the therapeutic relationship (*see* Book 4, Chapter 2) is a high priority.

In some instances people with mental health problems may be using substances that are exacerbating their mental health problem, yet they are not actually dependent on the substance. Brief interventions (*see* Book 4, Chapter 8) in this setting can still be effective at changing substance use.[21]

Brief interventions

With Maria's story from above, an opportunity has emerged for an initial brief intervention and motivational interviewing. Brief interventions[11] are designed specifically for primary care and involve a few minutes of information and counselling for people with non-dependent (but nevertheless hazardous) levels of substance use,

The GP could help Maria to check and some of the other adverse consequences of her cannabis use, as well as the longer-term respiratory and other problems from the tobacco. There is a range of ways the GP could help her through the process, including some counselling about quitting techniques, nicotine replacement, and other medications to help with the cannabis withdrawal, and perhaps getting her to look at some alternative meaningful activities during the day.

Do what is possible given the individual's readiness for change and insight

However, even in the situation where she is not ready for change, the GP can still help Maria in a number of ways. The important thing is to maintain a long-term outlook, act opportunistically, do whatever is possible that will help Maria maintain her health and wait for other opportunities regarding her comorbidity. For example, the GP or primary health team can do the following.
➤ Attend to Maria's physical health needs. We have good evidence that people with psychosis have significantly increased all-cause mortality.[22] General

physical health can be maintained through standard primary care measures, such as cervical screening, immunisation, identification of and attending to other cardiovascular risks, such as hypertension and hyperlipidaemia.

➤ Attend to aspects of her psychiatric care that do not require as much commitment from the individual, such as ensuring her depo-antipsychotics are given; that her mental state is monitored, and early deteriorations are detected and acted on before she becomes very unwell.

Harm reduction

A range of strategies can be implemented where readiness for change is limited while the person is continuing to use alcohol or other substances (*see* Chapter 15).

For example, if the person continues to use alcohol to a harmful level then thiamine supplementation, advice about avoiding drinking in particularly high-risk situations (driving, swimming), about adequate contraception, the use of condoms and safer sex are all options that reduce the adverse outcomes associated with risky drinking.

If the person is continuing to inject substances, advice about accessing sterile clean injecting equipment, not sharing equipment, lower-risk injection sites and technique, moving to less harmful routes of administration (such as smoking or snorting or ingesting), about not injecting alone, and about the availability of human immunodeficiency virus (HIV) post-exposure prophylaxis will reduce the harms associated with the use.

Structured problem-solving

People will come to their general practice with a range of problems. Not all of these are due to organic *disease*. 'Sickness' can be conceptualised in the following ways.[23]

➤ **Diseases** – discernible as physically 'real', with tissue changes able to be seen, valid even in the absence of illness, and amoral.

➤ **Illnesses** – an experience that may be linked to a disease, a social manifestation, a role, that may vary with respect to the disease they represent, and which may be judged morally.

➤ **Predicaments** – the complex of psychosocial ramifications, contacts, meanings and ascriptions, diffuse and multifactorial, inherently unstable, painful regardless of the presence of illness or disease, and highly morally and ethically loaded.[23]

Most of the psychosocial problems that individuals bring to general practitioners are predicament-related. If they also experience problems with their mental health and substance use, their capacity to logically problem solve will be diminished (*see* Chapter 8). The above categorisation of what we face in general practice is handy for sorting through appropriate response options.

Structured problem-solving is a brief counselling technique for helping individuals sort out their predicaments. The steps are outlined as:[24]

➤ Step 1: What is the problem/goal?

➤ Step 2: List all possible solutions.

➤ Step 3: Assess each possible solution.

➤ Step 4: Choose the 'best' or most practical solution.
➤ Step 5: Plan how to carry out the best solution.
➤ Step 6: Review progress and be pleased with any progress.[24]

While simple at first glance, the process is surprisingly effective. Structured problem-solving can be taught in general practice and can be effective, not only with generic predicament-related problems but also in the management of people with mild to moderate degrees of depression.[25] A work-sheet for using with individuals is available at the Black Dog Institute website: www.blackdoginstitute.org.au/docs/16. ProblemStructuredProblemSolvingexercise.pdf.

Motivational interviewing

Motivational interviewing (*see* Book 4, Chapter 7) is a person-centred technique designed to bring about behaviour change through developing incongruence in the individual.[26] The clinician explores the individual's lifestyle, stresses and day-to-day substance use. The perceived benefits of the behaviour, then any down-sides associated with the substance use, are examined. The clinician helps the individual look at the longer-term goals and draws the individual towards some of the incongruence between his/her longer-term goals and their current behaviour. The technique works on the individual's ambivalence but avoids confrontation.

While used largely in the context of substance use, motivational interviewing is effective in a range of clinical settings involving behaviour change.[28]

Motivational interviewing can be a very useful tool in the primary care setting. One of the benefits of general practice or primary care is that the clinician often has several opportunities to address the particular problematic behaviour – and can pace the intervention accordingly and take advantage of opportunities arising from presentations that might be linked with the behaviour.

Brief cognitive and behavioural interventions

There is a range of evidence-based cognitive behaviourally based interventions that can be applied in the primary care or general practice setting. Brief interventions (*see* Book 4, Chapter 15; Book 5, Chapter 14) for moderate or high-risk substance use, motivational interviewing, structured problem-solving are already described above.

Advice regarding slow breathing exercises, relaxation training, activity scheduling, sleep hygiene, advice regarding aerobic exercise, as well as the interventions described above, can be used.

In addition more extended programmes of cognitive therapy and exposure therapy can be delivered in the primary care setting not only by general practitioners but also by psychologists and specifically trained nurse therapists or other counsellors (*see* Book 4, Chapter 10; Book 5, Chapters 11, 12, 13).[28]

Pharmacotherapies

General practitioners are in a good position to prescribe indicated medications for a range of mental disorders (antidepressants, antipsychotics, mood stabilisers, anxiolytics in limited circumstances) and substance use-related problems (anti-craving medications such as naltrexone and acamprosate for alcohol dependence, substitution therapies for opioid and nicotine dependence).

Having most or all medications prescribed by the one prescriber or at least the one service reduces the risk of poly-pharmacy, unforeseen drug interactions and redundant prescribing (*see* Book 5, Chapter 13).

Working with families

The work of primary care with families is fairly unique (*see* Chapter 2; Book 5, Chapters 7, 14). While for the most part this work is with individual members of the family, there are unique opportunities that are not generally available to the specialist service.

There are confidentiality issues to be considered. However, if free flow of information is consented to, the primary care clinician can use information from other members of the family to triangulate information given by the individual about their mental state and substance use.

In addition, members of the family of an individual experiencing mental health–substance use problems also experience hardships associated with their family member's mental health–substance use. Members of the primary care team can assist these family members with finding the most appropriate response to the problem. At times this can set up conflicts of interest, or at least perceptions of such, but on the whole these can be reduced by having different professionals work with the individual members of the family.

Finally, enlisting the support of family members to help with responding to the person experiencing mental health–substance use problems[29] can improve outcomes. The primary care team has an important role in this enlistment and support of family members.

REFERRAL TO SERVICES EXTERNAL TO PRIMARY CARE

Referral to specialist services is indicated in various situations, assuming that there are specialist services available to refer to who will accept the individual. The way specialist services are arranged varies from country to country and area to area. Selecting the most appropriate referral pathway is sometimes problematic. In those health systems where the addiction services are separated from mental health/psychiatric services, either specialist service can try to deflect the referral to the alternative one. In arrangements where the two types of service are better integrated, this makes the referrals from primary care easier. If the GP is working in a setting with a healthy private sector, referral into the private system for individuals who are insured is an additional option. There is no substitute for local knowledge in this context.

However, there seems to be some common threads to the referral pathways in different developed countries with integrated health systems.

Generally speaking, the specialist mental health services will be the service to refer to where:

➤ the person is actively psychotic
➤ there are major concerns about the safety of the individual due to risk of self-harm

➤ there are major concerns about the safety of others due to the behaviour of the individual.

If the individual is *not* psychotic and *not* a risk to themselves or to others it is less likely that specialist mental health services (at least publicly funded ones) will have the capacity to help by accepting the referral. Again there will always be variations and in some health systems there will be adequate access to specialist services for complex individuals other than the limited range above.

As far as referrals to alcohol and drug services are concerned, consider referral in the following situations.

➤ Serious substance dependence is identified, requiring a multidisciplinary approach. This is the case particularly with poly-drug dependence, where dependence has been present for several years; where there are high levels of dysfunction and when the individual is socially isolated.

➤ Complicated detoxification is anticipated. The most worrying detoxification is from alcohol. Generally, individuals with the following characteristics are likely to require inpatient admission for detoxification:
  — those with significant physical comorbidities
  — those who are already acutely ill, e.g. with pneumonia, dehydration, or trauma
  — those who are drinking more than 80 g of pure alcohol per day
  — those who are over 30 years of age.

➤ There is lack of treatment response despite several attempts using a variety of techniques/interventions.

KEY POINT 10.3

Communication between all treating services/professionals is often a significant problem. A number of elements should be agreed to early on in the treatment cycle:
- contact details of all treating professionals
- arrangements for shared care describing the roles of each service/professionals
- case conferences should be held as required or in on a regular timetable. These can occur face to face or alternatively by teleconference
- emergency plans/contact details for those professionals involved in care.

At times specialist treatment services can support GPs by taking responsibility for changes to treatment with which the individual may not be entirely happy (e.g. restricted access to drugs or dependence such as opioids or benzodiazepines). The same would apply to mandated treatments under various mental health legislations if these are in place in the particular relevant jurisdiction. This enables the GP to maintain a positive therapeutic relationship (*see* Book 4, Chapter 2) that might otherwise be jeopardised.

More formal arrangements for service coordination should be developed by regional primary care and specialist care bureaucracies to ensure that these types of arrangements are streamlined and institutional blocks are addressed.

SUPERVISION AND PEER SUPPORT FOR GENERAL PRACTITIONERS

GPs with a special interest in this area have particular peer support and supervision needs. There are a number of patient, clinician and contextual factors unique to working in the mental health–substance use fields that necessitate supervision or peer support. While these concepts are familiar to psychiatry and psychology, and the counselling fields, they are less accepted in general practice (*see* Book 1, Chapter 10).

Peer support can be seen to have three main functions:[30]

➤ **Normative** – focusing on ensuring that the general performance of the clinician is 'normal' compared with peers.

➤ **Formative** – where knowledge and skills can be developed and improved.

➤ **Restorative** – where clinicians gain support and encouragement.

There is a range of activities that can serve these peer support functions, although current professional development and peer support activities tend to mostly focus on the formative skills development functions.[31] For any of the three functions above to be adequately addressed, the activities need to be specifically designed and carried out. Balint groups, for example, focus more on restorative functions.[32] Group activities if properly planned are cost effective, can be powerful normative influences and can provide excellent support. An atmosphere of trust is important; in addition, the guidance of a professional external to the group and the immediate 'culture' of the participants in order to challenge group norms is an important safety measure. More information on Balint groups can be accessed at http://americanbalintsociety.org/.

Other types of activities include regular direct observation, reviews of video or audiotaped consultations, and indirect case reviews using the case notes as an aide-memoire. These can be done randomly or in a selected manner. These types of activity can be done either as one to one activities or in groups. Where distance is an issue in remote areas, such activities can be done by telephone or video-teleconference with relative ease using modern technologies.

> **KEY POINT 10.4**
>
> Primary care services and general practices if they have significant mental health–substance use workloads (and which ones don't?) need to consider peer support and supervision as an intrinsic element of their clinical governance frameworks. This is both to enhance quality of service and to support and protect professionals.

CONCLUSIONS

General practice and primary care allow a long-term opportunistic approach to people with mental health–substance use. There is a range of interventions that can be used in the primary care setting. GPs and other primary care professionals also have a unique opportunity to work with families of people experiencing mental health–substance use problems, even if the individual is disengaged.

Finally, working alongside individuals with this range of problems can be taxing and has some associated risks. Peer support and supervision are important activities that help to ensure that both clinicians and individuals remain safe and services are optimised.

REFERENCES

1 Starfield B. *Primary Care Balancing Health Needs, Services and Technology.* New York: Oxford University Press; 1998. p. 29.

2 Bourdon KH, Rae DS, Locke BZ, *et al.* Estimating the prevalence of mental disorders in U.S. adults from the Epidemiologic Catchment Area Survey. *Public Health Reports.* 1992; **107**: 663–8.

3 Harvard University. National Comorbidity Survey: NCS-R 12-month prevalence estimates. Available at: www.hcp.med.harvard.edu/ncs/ftpdir/table_ncsr_12monthprevgenderxage. pdf (accessed 1 July 2010).

4 Australian Bureau of Statistics Canberra. *Australian National Survey of Mental Health and Wellbeing*; 2007. Available at: www.ausstats.abs.gov.au/ausstats/subscriber.nsf/0/6AE6DA 447F985FC2CA2574EA00122BD6/$File/43260_2007.pdf (accessed 1 July 2010).

5 Hickie I, Koschera A, Davenport T, *et al.* Comorbidity of common mental disorders and alcohol or other substance misuse in Australian general practice in SPHERE: a national depression initiative. *Medical Journal of Australia.* 2001; **165**: S31.

6 Teesson M. Chapter background: causes, prevention and treatment of comorbidity. In: Teesson M, Burns L, and National Drug and Alcohol Research Centre, editors. *National Comorbidity Project.* Canberra, ACT: Commonwealth Department of Health and Aged Care; 2001. p. 8.

7 Goldberg D, Blackwell B. Psychiatric illness in general practice: a detailed study using a new method of case identification. *British Medical Journal.* 1970; **1**: 439–43.

8 Sartorius N, Ustun B, Costa e Silva J, *et al.* An international study of psychological problems in primary care. *Archives of General Psychiatry.* 1993; **50**: 819–24.

9 Fucito LM, Gomes BS. Murnion B, *et al.* General practitioners' diagnostic skills and referral practices in managing patients with drug and alcohol-related health problems: implications for medical training and education programmes. *Drug and Alcohol Review.* 2003; **22**: 117–24.

10 Rehm J, Room R, Monteiro M, *et al.* Alcohol as a risk factor for global burden of disease. *European Addiction Research.* 2003; **9**: 157–64.

11 Babor TF, Higgins-Biddle JC. *Brief Intervention for Hazardous and Harmful Drinking: a manual for use in primary care.* Geneva: World Health Organization; 2001. Available at: http://whqlibdoc.who.int/hq/2001/WHO_MSD_MSB_01.6b.pdf (accessed 1 July 2010).

12 Andrews G, Issakidis C, Slade T. The clinical significance of mental disorders. In: Teesson M, Burns L, National Drug and Alcohol Research Centre, editors. *National Comorbidity Project.* Canberra, ACT: Commonwealth Department of Health and Aged Care; 2001.

13 Goldberg D, Steele JJ, Johnson A, *et al.* Ability of primary care physicians to make accurate ratings of psychiatric symptoms. *Archives of General Psychiatry.* 1982; **39**: 829–33.

14 Goldberg D, Steele JJ, Smith C. Teaching psychiatric interview techniques to family doctors. *Acta Psychiatrica Scandinavica.* 1982; **62**(Suppl.): S41–7.

15 Goldberg D, Steele JJ, Smith C, *et al.* Training family doctors to recognise psychiatric illness with increased accuracy. *Lancet.* 1982; **3**: 521–4.

16 McCabe D, Holmwood C. *Comorbidity of Mental Disorders and Substance Use in General Practice.* Canberra, ACT: Australian Government Department of Health and Ageing; 2001.

17 De Maeseneer J, Deveugele M, Derese A, *et al.* Consultation length in general practice: a cross-sectional study in six European countries. *British Medical Journal.* 2002; **325**: 472.

18 Britt H, Valenti L, Miller G. Time for care. Length of general practice consultations in Australia. *Australian Family Physician.* 2002; **31**: 876–80.

19 Prochaska JO, DiClemente CC. Trans-theoretical therapy: toward a more integrative model of change. *Psychotherapy: Theory, Research and Practice.* 1982; **19**: 276–88.

20 Miller P, Thomas S, Mallin R. Patient attitudes towards self-report and biomarker alcohol screening by primary care physicians. *Alcohol and Alcoholism.* 2006; **41**: 306–10.

21 Kavanagh D, Young R, Saunders JB, *et al.* A brief intervention for comorbidity of substance abuse and mental disorder. *Australian and New Zealand Journal of Psychiatry.* 2002; **36**: A20.

22 Lambert T. The medical care of people with psychosis. *Medical Journal of Australia.* 2009; **190**: 171–2.

23 Davis CT. The components of sickness: diseases, illnesses and predicaments. *Lancet.* 1979; **10**: 1008–10.

24 Andrews G, Hunt C. Treatments that work in anxiety disorders. *Medical Journal of Australia Practice Essentials.* 1998; **1**: 26–31. Available at: www.mja.com.au/public/mentalhealth/articles/andrews/andrews.html (accessed 1 July 2010).

25 Mynors-Wallis LM, Gath DH, Day A, *et al.* Randomised controlled trial of problem solving treatment, antidepressant medication, and combined treatment for major depression in primary care. *British Medical Journal.* 2000; **320**: 26–30.

26 Miller WR, Rollnick S. *Motivational Interviewing: preparing people to change.* New York: Guilford Press; 2002.

27 Rubak S. Motivational interviewing: a systematic review and meta-analysis. *British Journal of General Practice.* 2005; **55**: 305–12.

28 Jackson Bowers E, Holmwood C, McCabe D. Models of primary health care psychotherapy and counselling. *Report for the Commonwealth Department of Health and Aged Care and the Access to Allied Health Task Group.* Primary Mental Health Care Australian Resource Centre Department of General Practice, Flinders University, November 2001. Available at: http://pandora.nla.gov.au/pan/35831/20030911-0000/som.flinders.edu.au/FUSA/PARC/Alliedhealthlitrev.pdf (accessed 1 July 2010).

29 Clark RE. Family support and substance use outcomes for people with mental illness and substance use disorders. *Association for Health Services Research Meeting.* 1999; **16**: 393.

30 Proctor B. Supervision: a co-operative exercise in accountability. In: Marken M, Payne M, editors. *Enabling and Ensuring.* Leicester: Leicester National Youth Bureau and Council for Education and Training in Youth and Community Work; 1986. pp. 21–3.

31 Jackson Bowers E, Holmwood C. *General Practitioners' Peer Support Needs in Managing Consumers' Mental Health Problems: a literature review and needs analysis.* Primary Mental Health Care Australian Resource Centre; 2002. Available at: http://dspace.flinders.edu.au/dspace/bitstream/2328/3204/1/peersupport.pdf (accessed 1 July 2010).

32 Samuel O. How doctors learn in a Balint group. *Family Practice.* 1989; **6**: 108.

TO LEARN MORE

- **Black Dog Institute**: www.blackdoginstitute.org.au/docs/16.ProblemStructuredProblemSolvingexercise.pdf
- **American Balint Society**: http://americanbalintsociety.org/
- **Australian Drug Information Network**: www.adin.com.au/content.asp?Document_ID=74

- Gordon A. *Comorbidity of Mental Disorders and Substance Use: a brief guide for the primary care clinician*. Canberra, ACT: Department of Health; 2008. www.nationaldrugstrategy.gov. au/internet/drugstrategy/Publishing.nsf/content/mono71
- Mills KL, Deady M, Proudfoot H, *et al. Guidelines on the Management of Co-occurring Alcohol and other Drug and Mental Health Conditions in Alcohol and other Drug Treatment Settings*. Australia: National Drug and Alcohol Research Centre University of New South Wales Sydney, Australia. www.med.unsw.edu.au/NDARCWeb.nsf/page/Comorbidity+Guidelines

Mental health–substance use: presenting together in primary care – the practical challenge

Hugh M Campbell

INTRODUCTION

The evidence base for mental health–substance use has a largely mental health perspective, and much that is written has only indirect relevance to primary care. The evidence base for assessment and treatment of mental health–substance use in primary care, therefore, is limited.

The personal relationship between general practitioner (GP) and the individual is unique and has been the subject of theoretical interest for many years.[1] GPs come to know the presenting individual (within the context of a family structure), as a human being who brings a unique and meaningful story. Diagnoses, discussions about service provision, and consideration of need, important as they are, are secondary to a sense of the human personality of the individual. This is especially true when considering mental health–substance use. Experience has taught this author a great deal and some authentic examples will be described later (names and some details have been altered to preserve anonymity).

REFLECTIVE PRACTICE EXERCISE 11.1

Time: 40 minutes

Reflect on a patient you may have been involved with recently who was experiencing mental health–substance use problems. Consider the learning that took place for you. How might this be of value when working with other individuals?

Important aspects of the general practitioner and individual contract

These include:

➤ general medical services (holistic care)
➤ continuity of care 24 hours a day (though responsibility may be delegated)
➤ open access free at the point of need

> GP consultations average six minutes but may be longer
> reliance on attached professionals, e.g. practice counsellor, nurse, or non-attached member of mental health team, or drug and alcohol team
> avenues of referral to a variety of specialists.

Primary care embraces the psychotherapeutic view that each of us is on an escalator of ascending or descending mental health. The same is true for the use of substances, from abstinence to recreational, hazardous, problematic or dependent use. Employing an appropriate care plan can help chart the progress of an individual experiencing mental health–substance use problems.[2]

Mental health problems may present in a wide range of ways in primary care

These include:
> schizophrenia[3]
> psychosis
> mood disorders[4]
> bipolar disorder[5]
> anxiety[6]
> personality disorder (particularly borderline and antisocial disorders)[7,8]
> obsessive–compulsive disorder[9]
> post-traumatic stress disorder (particularly sexual abuse in both women and men)[10]
> learning disability/difficulty[6]
> eating disorders[11]
> dementia.[12]

Use of substances

Use of the following substances is common:
> alcohol
> cannabis
> stimulants
> benzodiazepines
> nicotine
> opiates, especially heroin
> hallucinogens
> solvents.

Non-substance addiction, e.g. gambling, hyper-sexuality, or relationship co-dependency may also feature in the context of mental health–substance use.

Mental health problems and substance use is complex; and so is the relationship between them. Rational linear thinking, upon which most medical assessment and treatment relies, is of limited value, and has been one of the reasons for the lack of progress in planning service provision for many individuals in this group. Other styles, such as complexity thinking, which is based on chaos theory, can bring a richer understanding and yield more fruitful solutions.[13–15]

Possible relationships between substance use and mental health include the following:[16]
> a primary illness precipitating or leading to substance use
> substance use worsening or altering the course of a psychiatric illness,

e.g. intoxication and/or substance dependence leading to psychological symptoms
- substance use and/or withdrawal leading to psychiatric symptoms or illness
- substances (especially alcohol, cannabis, stimulants and hallucinogens) producing psychotic symptoms without mental illness.

Why may those with mental health problems use substances?[16]

REFLECTIVE PRACTICE EXERCISE 11.2

Time: 5 minutes

Take time to reflect. Can you add anything to the following list?

People with mental health problems may use substances for the following reasons.
- To escape, to get high.
- Increased availability in poor city areas to decrease social isolation (social drift hypothesis).
- Availability in prisons and psychiatric units.
- Self-medication of anxiety or depression.
- Some stimulants counteract the extra-pyramidal effects of antipsychotic medication.
- Perhaps there is a common genetic susceptibility for both conditions?

Substance use by individuals with mental health problems is associated with significantly poorer outcomes, including:[16]
- worsening psychiatric symptoms
- increased rates of self-harm/suicidal behaviour
- increased rates of violence[17,18]
- poor medication compliance
- increased rates of blood-borne virus infections
- higher service use
- higher rates of homelessness
- high incidence of physical problems, including complications relating to smoking, nutrition and infections, e.g. tuberculosis.

What can primary care offer the individual experiencing mental health–substance use and complex needs?

SELF-ASSESSMENT EXERCISE 11.1

Time: 10 minutes

Consider yourself as a user of the service:
- What might you expect/hope for in terms of service provision?
- Why would this be important for you?

Primary care can offer the individual experiencing mental health–substance use and complex needs the following:

➤ continuity of care
➤ holistic general medical services
➤ enhanced services for coexisting physical problems
➤ coordination between services
➤ crisis intervention
➤ containment
➤ care for family/carers
➤ advocacy
➤ medication review
➤ help with housing and benefits
➤ risk assessment.

WHAT ARE THE ISSUES FOR PRIMARY CARE DEALING WITH THE INDIVIDUAL EXPERIENCING MENTAL HEALTH–SUBSTANCE USE?

Issues include the following:

➤ assessment
➤ identifying needs
➤ risks for the individual, including self-harm, violence, neglect and child protection[17–19]
➤ risk for the practitioner, including risk of assault
➤ prescribing issues, use of unfamiliar drugs which may attract audit/clinical governance/or media attention
➤ consent
➤ confidentiality
➤ lack of support
➤ inadequate access to other services
➤ referral procedures
➤ housing issues[20]
➤ time commitment for multi-agency meetings.

Despite this, the primary care practitioner is ideally suited to coordinate and support the care of complex mental health–substance use needs and may often be able to provide well-organised, shrewd treatment for those who do not meet criteria for other services or have fallen out/been excluded from treatment for arbitrary reasons, e.g. non-attendance of appointments.

Assessment

Given the 10-minute time constraint, the following is a menu of approaches that may be relevant.[21]

➤ Encourage individuals to tell the story their way (narrative approach).
➤ Establishing chronology and interrelationship of mental health problems with substance use.
➤ Ensure an adequate mental health assessment including mood, anxiety level,

screening for psychotic symptoms, vulnerability, safety, risk to self and others, violence/forensic potential.

➤ Consider use of depression, self-harm and violence-rating instruments.[17,19,22]

➤ Enquire about details of substance use: types of substance, amounts, frequency, routes of administration, history of use, context of use, dependence including indication of severity.[23,24]

➤ Assessment of other problems, physical (including blood-borne virus infection), social, criminal, housing, family.[25]

➤ Liaise with other services to complete the picture.

KEY POINT 11.1

Assessment requires great skill, flexibility, focus and practice.

It is not possible to present every case scenario that might be met during practice as they are all varied and complex. However, the examples below might offer a feel for the GP's position in practice and the decisions that often need to be taken. An experienced GP can offer a range of clinical knowledge and skills. See the 'To learn more' section of this chapter for useful references to develop one's knowledge and understanding further.

Case study 11.1

Irene, 24, uses heroin, and is from another town. She presents for the first time at the end of a busy morning surgery. Irene wishes to register and tells you that a close family member died in tragic circumstances in your locality a week ago. Irene presents as tearful, distressed and has objective signs of opiate withdrawal. She is staying temporarily with relatives. Irene gives you a prescription slip from her GP with evidence that she takes regular:

- diazepam 30 mg daily
- fluoxetine 20 mg daily
- olanzapine 10 mg daily
- dihydrocodeine 240 mg daily.

The last Irene takes for chronic sciatica. Irene tells you that she is also taking methadone mixture 80 mL daily, and that her last dose was 48 hours ago. She is hepatitis C positive and smells faintly of alcohol. Attempts to contact her GP, drug, or mental health professional, or the local addiction psychiatrist prove impossible. You discuss the case with the local duty drug worker.

SELF-ASSESSMENT EXERCISE 11.2

Time: 10 minutes
- What are the primary issues here?
- How would you deal with them?

What are the issues here and how do you deal with them?

The main problem is that you know very little about Irene. Her presentation, and limited information about prescribing, suggests that she is at risk, both because of her mental health history and probable substance use.

No one else is available to make a more detailed assessment so clinical responsibility remains with you.

SELF-ASSESSMENT EXERCISE 11.3

Time: 5 minutes
Consider:
- What are your feelings?
- How might you respond?

You feel professionally isolated. This could take time to sort out.

SELF-ASSESSMENT EXERCISE 11.4

Time: 10 minutes
What are the possible approaches in this situation?

What are the possible approaches in this situation?

Continue to seek further confirmatory information. Try to phone her GP again. Encourage Irene to offer more details of her drug service, mental health contacts and pharmacy where she collects her methadone.

Pressure your local drug service to seek information and request an early drug assessment. This is a potential service transfer.

Attempt drug testing; urine testing sticks may show positive for opiates but this may be unhelpful because you know she has taken dihydrocodeine. Drug urine testing may take several days even for an urgent request. It may be possible to access emergency toxicology, a service normally reserved for individuals from criminal justice. It proved possible to access the latter, and Irene's urine showed positive to heroin, methadone and codeine.

Consequently, Irene commenced on a titration dose of methadone, starting at 30 mL daily and increasing by 10 mL daily, with regular face to face contact either with you or a drug worker. She was also issued with a three-day supply of her other medication.

Irene was seen daily and one week later, after the family member's funeral, was stabilised on 60 mL methadone daily and was planning to stay in your district.

Case study 11.2

Andrew is single, 29 and unemployed. He moved into your area and wishes to register. He came with a letter from his GP saying that Andrew was heroin dependent but had managed to stabilise his habit on dihydrocodeine (DHC) 600 mg daily. He saw no one for check-ups apart from his GP, never had urine screens and was prescribed on a monthly basis. He also had a history of severe anxiety and found the opiates helped this.

SELF-ASSESSMENT EXERCISE 11.5

Time: 10 minutes
- How would you assess Andrew?
- How would you manage his opiate prescribing?

How do we assess Andrew, and how are we going to manage his opiate prescribing?

It is important to build a trusting relationship with Andrew and engage in his care. A review of his treatment with the offer of a more skilled assessment by a drug worker or community psychiatric nurse would be helpful. There is a need to consider Andrew's use of other illicit agents. Drug use screening is beneficial. Consider with Andrew changing short-acting DHC for a longer acting opiate, either methadone or buprenorphine.

If successful, you could greatly improve his treatment. Andrew opted to reduce his DHC, which was prescribed on a weekly basis, and currently he takes just 60 mg daily, planning to stop altogether. A full answer to this is given elsewhere.[26]

COLLABORATIVE TREATMENT APPROACHES BETWEEN PRIMARY AND SECONDARY CARE

Some of the issues are illustrated with examples.

Case study 11.3

Paul, 52, was on diamorphine prescription for many years from addiction psychiatry for heroin dependency. He also has low-level psychosis. He presents infrequently for support and prescriptions of sulpiride, which relieve his psychotic thoughts. Three months previously Paul had been admitted for a residential detoxification, which he completed successfully, although within days of leaving rehabilitation he relapsed on heroin in low dosage and also started to drink heavily. Paul started to inject about £30 of heroin daily, and was drinking 2 litres of cider daily. After reassessment by the specialist service he was started on methadone 50 mL daily and produced several clean screens. However, his alcohol intake continued to escalate. After three months he was drinking 4–6 litres of cider daily. Paul wanted a community alcohol detoxification and also wanted help to quit smoking (currently 40 cigarettes daily).

SELF-ASSESSMENT EXERCISE 11.6

Time: 10 minutes
- What are the issues here?
- How can you best help Paul?

What are the issues here? How can you best help Andrew?

Phone liaison with Paul's specialist drugs worker is essential. A more detailed alcohol assessment confirmed that he was now alcohol dependent and probably needed an alcohol detoxification. His feelings of failure after relapse, shortly after an opiate detoxification, might be relevant, and the fact that Paul is on a methadone prescription increases the clinical complexity. Drinking at this level while on methadone is hazardous and needs to be explained to Paul.

Paul successfully detoxed from alcohol using a reducing-dose chlordiazepoxide reduction regime with full support from his community psychiatric nurse. After several weeks of alcohol abstinence Paul was referred to the practice nurse to prepare for a 'QUIT' attempt using nicotine replacement. However, this was less successful and he was later referred to the local specialist smoking cessation service.

Case study 11.4

Cheryl, 25, came to your locality for drug rehabilitation in 2003. Her drugs of use were heroin, amphetamines and benzodiazepines. She also suffered from a range of severe but ill-defined mental health problems, but in rehabilitation she had no contact with the local mental health service. After successfully detoxing, she left rehabilitation but resettled in your area. The following three years were stormy with several mental health admissions, often with sectioning. She relapsed on heroin and was eventually reassessed by addiction psychiatry and started again on methadone 60 mL daily. She had a comprehensive mental health review and was given the following diagnoses:
- borderline personality disorder
- recurrent depression
- chronic psychosis
- learning difficulties
- adult attention deficit hyperactivity disorder.

Sheryl also had hypothyroidism, chronic low back pain with sciatica and chronic hepatitis C. Her other medications included:

- fluoxetine 20 mg daily
- risperidone 6 mg daily
- thyroid replacement
- diazepam 10 mg nocte
- modafinil.

Over the last three years she has been supported by a community psychiatric nurse, complex needs drug worker and you. Each sees Sheryl regularly. You see her monthly for brief monitoring and issue of her medication apart from her methadone (dispensed daily). The non-opiate part of the prescription is issued weekly. There have been no episodes of self-harm for some months and no inpatient treatment for over two years.

Comment

This method of support with severe mental health, substance use and other medical problems seems to be working well. The key is that each member of the support team has a well-defined role within a wider care plan. The community psychiatric nurse and complex needs professional have their own individual care plans that define their responsibility. Borderline individuals have particular difficulty with relationships and this arrangement holds well with good communication between professionals.

CONCLUSION

The above illustrations demonstrate how diverse and complex mental health–substance use problems can be in a primary care setting. Only those with severe mental health disturbance or problematic substance use get the intensity and degree of specialism required for their treatment from an addiction psychiatry team (integrated treatment). A common alternative to this is parallel treatment from a mental health team and/or substance use service. Some of those who fail to engage with secondary care, and most of the individuals experiencing less severe mental health disturbance and substance use, become the responsibility of the primary care practitioner. The skills to carry this responsibility are wide and varied. The evidence base for treatment of mental health–substance use in primary care is flimsy as most evidence relates to other settings. Finally, the guidance of Linehan (for the dialectic treatment of borderline individuals) is relevant to the general practitioner: *'be oriented to change yet oriented to acceptance, nurturing but benevolently demanding, unwaveringly centred yet compassionately flexible'.*[27]

REFERENCES

1 Innes A, Campion D, Griffiths F. Complex consultations and the 'edge of chaos'. *British Journal of General Practice*. 2005; **55**: 47–52.

2 Department of Health. *Models of Care for Substance Misuse Treatment: promoting quality, efficiency and effectiveness in drug misuse treatment services.* London: HMSO; 2002.

3 National Institute for Health and Clinical Excellence. *Schizophrenia (update): core interventions in the treatment and management of schizophrenia in adults in primary and secondary care.* NICE guideline 82. London: NIHCE; 2009. Available at: www.nice.org.uk/cg82 (accessed 2 July 2010).

4 National Institute for Health and Clinical Excellence. *Depression: management of depression in primary and secondary care.* NICE guideline 23. London: NIHCE; 2004. Available at: www.nice.org.uk/CG90 (accessed 2 July 2010).

5 National Institute for Health and Clinical Excellence. *Bipolar Disorder: the management of bipolar disorder in adults, children and adolescents in primary and secondary care.* NICE guideline 38. London: NIHCE; 2006. Available at: www.nice.org.uk/cg38 (accessed 5 July 2010).

6 National Institute for Health and Clinical Excellence. *Attention Deficit Hyperactivity Disorder (ADHD): methyl phenidate, atomoxetine and dexamfetamine (review).* NICE guideline 72. London: NIHCE; 2006. Available at: www.nice.org.uk/cg72 (accessed 5 July 2010).

7 National Institute for Health and Clinical Excellence. *Antisocial Personality Disorder: treatment, management and prevention.* NICE guideline 77. London: NIHCE; 2009. Available at: www.nice.org.uk/cg77 (accessed 5 July 2010).

8 National Institute for Health and Clinical Excellence. *Borderline Personality Disorder: treatment and management.* NICE guideline 78. London: NIHCE; 2009. Available at: www.nice.org.uk/cg78 (accessed 5 July 2010).

9 National Institute for Health and Clinical Excellence. *Obsessive-compulsive Disorder: core interventions in the treatment of obsessive-compulsive disorder and body dysmorphic disorder.* NICE guideline 31. London: NIHCE; 2005. Available at: www.nice.org.uk/cg31 (accessed 5 July 2010).

10 National Institute for Health and Clinical Excellence. *Post-traumatic Stress Disorder (PTSD): the management of PTSD in adults and children in primary and secondary care.* NICE guideline 26. London: NIHCE; 2005. Available at: www.nice.org.uk/cg26 (accessed 5 July 2010).

11 National Institute for Health and Clinical Excellence. *Eating Disorders: core interventions in the treatment of anorexia nervosa, bulimia nervosa and related eating disorders.* NICE guideline 9. London: NIHCE; 2004. Available at: www.nice.org.uk/cg9 (accessed 5 July 2010).

12 National Institute for Health and Clinical Excellence. *Dementia: supporting people with dementia and their carers in health and social care.* NICE guideline 42. London: NIHCE; 2006. Available at: www.nice.org.uk/cg42 (accessed 5 July 2010).

13 Hassey A. Complexity and the clinical encounter. In: Sweeney K, Griffith F, editors. *Complexity and Healthcare: an introduction.* Oxford: Radcliffe Medical Press; 2002. pp. 59–74.

14 Holt T. Clinical knowledge, chaos and complexity. In: Sweeney K, Griffith F, editors. *Complexity and Healthcare: an introduction.* Oxford: Radcliffe Medical Press; 2002. pp. 35–73.

15 Whittle J, Bosworth H. Studying complexity is complex. *Journal of General Internal Medicine.* 2007; **22**(Suppl. 3): 379–81.

16 Gerada C. Drug misuse and co-morbid illness: 'dual diagnosis'. *Royal College of General Practitioners Guide to the Management of Substance Misuse in Primary Care.* London: Royal College of General Practitioners; 2005. pp. 317–31.

17 Soyka M. Substance misuse, psychiatric disorder and violent and disturbed behaviour. *British Journal of Psychiatry.* 2000; **176**: 345–50.

18 National Institute for Health and Clinical Excellence. *Violence: the short-term management of disturbed/violent behaviour in in-patient psychiatric settings and emergency departments.* NICE guideline 25. London: NIHCE; 2005. Available at: www.nice.org.uk/cg25 (accessed 5 July 2010)

19 National Institute for Health and Clinical Excellence. *Self-harm: the short-term physical and psychological management and secondary prevention of self-harm in primary and secondary care.* NICE guideline 16. London: NIHCE; 2004. Available at: www.nice.org.uk/cg16 (accessed 5 July 2010).

20 Wright N. Drug use and housing issues. *Royal College of General Practitioners Guide to the Management of Substance Misuse in Primary Care.* London: Royal College of General Practitioners; 2005. pp. 307–16.

21 Department of Health. *Mental Health Policy Implementation Guide: dual diagnosis good practice guide.* London: HMSO; 2002.

22 *Patient Health Questionnaire PHQ-9 for Depression*; 2006. Available at: www.depression-primarycare.org (accessed 5 July 2010).

23 National Institute for Health and Clinical Excellence. *Drug Misuse: opioid detoxification.* NICE guideline 52. London: NIHCE; 2007. Available at: www.nice.org.uk/cg52 (accessed 5 July 2010).

24 National Institute for Health and Clinical Excellence. *Drug Misuse: psychosocial interventions.* NICE guideline 51. London: NIHCE; 2007. Available at: http://guidance.nice.org.uk/CG51 (accessed 5 July 2010).

25 Metabolic and lifestyle issues and severe mental illness: new connections to well-being? Expert consensus meeting, Dublin. *Journal of Psychopharmacology.* 2005; **19**: 118–22.

26 Campbell H. Dr Fixit on dual diagnosis. *Network.* 2008; **21**: 12–13.

27 Linehan M. *Cognitive-behavioural Treatment of Borderline Personality Disorder.* New York: Guildford; 1993. pp. 67, 109.

TO LEARN MORE

- Afuwape S. *Where are we with Dual Diagnosis (Substance Misuse and Mental Illness)? A review of the literature.* Rethink: Severe Mental Illness; 2003. Available at: www.rethink.org/document.rm?id=1927

- Crawford V, Crome I, Clancy C. Co-existing problems of mental health and substance misuse ('dual diagnosis'). *Journal of Drugs and Education: Prevention and Policy.* 2003; **10**: 1–74.

- Crawford V. Dual diagnosis: what does policy and research tell us? *Network.* 2008; **21**: 14–15.

- Patient UK *Dual Diagnosis (drug abuse with other psychiatric conditions)*; 2008. Available at: www.patient.co.uk/doctor/Dual-Diagnosis-(Drug-abuse-with-other-psychiatric-conditions).htm

- Royal College of Psychiatrists. *Dual Diagnosis Information Manual: extensive information for practitioners working in the field.* London: Royal College of Psychiatrists; 2002.

- Gerada C. Drug misuse and co-morbid illness: 'dual diagnosis'. In: *Royal College of General Practitioners Guide to the Management of Substance Misuse in Primary Care.* London: Royal College of General Practitioners; 2005. pp. 317–31.

- Lingford-Hughes A, Welch S, Nutt D. Evidence-based guidelines for the pharmacological management of substance misuse, addiction and comorbidity: recommendations from the British association for psychopharmacology. *Journal of Psychopharmacology.* 2004; **18**: 293–335.

CHAPTER 12

Integrated service and system planning debate

Brian R Rush and Louise Nadeau

INTRODUCTION

Historically, the design and deployment of publicly funded human services and supports (e.g. health, social, education, justice) have been compartmentalised to make them more targeted to the needs of specific populations, more manageable and, arguably, more accountable. This explains in large part the initial separation of substance use and mental health services (at least in North American and many other countries). This 'siloing' of services notwithstanding, the increasing complexity and intractability of a given problem domain contributes to a 'reverse pressure' to form various types of inter-organisational relationships and cross-sectoral strategies to better address people's needs. In some instances, these relationships evolve naturally, and often informally, at the community level. In other instances, they become mandated and structural solutions are dictated.

In this chapter we provide an update on the issues and challenges related to the integration of mental health and substance use services and systems. It is not our intention to be highly prescriptive; rather, our primary aims are to:

➤ review the rationale for better integration of these service delivery sectors
➤ identify key features of alternative models for improving integration and evaluating the benefits.

To set the stage for proper coverage of these topic areas we identify three foundational sub-topics that are critical to any concrete attempts towards better integration.

1 One must be clear regarding who is expected to benefit.
2 One must locate 'integration' within a broader design framework for mental health and substance use services, including those for people experiencing mental health–substance use disorders.
3 One must articulate the important distinction between integration at the service and system levels.

In conclusion, we briefly place this discourse within the context of the research literature on the effective components of treatment for substance use, mental health, and mental health–substance use disorders.

FOUNDATIONAL ELEMENTS FOR PLANNING AND EVALUATING INTEGRATION STRATEGIES
Who are the expected beneficiaries?

In the majority of best practice reviews to date (e.g. Substance Abuse and Mental Health Services Administration,[1] Health Canada[2]), the term concurrent or co-occurring 'disorders' is used to define the primary target population for improved integration of mental health and substance use services and systems. In an effort to be precise, those with mental health–substance use disorders typically refer to people meeting the criteria for both a substance use disorder and another mental disorder as defined by strict DSM-based or ICD-9 classification systems for psychiatric disorders. This approach offers many advantages, in particular for research and knowledge exchange (e.g. the development of clinical guidelines and identifying core clinical competencies). However, the relatively narrow definition of mental health–substance use may limit clinical practice. It may also present challenges for planning at a community systems level since it does not adequately embrace the large segment of the population that may either be 'sub-threshold' of these disorders, or at moderate to high risk of developing them. Further, people experiencing mental health–substance use disorders often experience many other health and social challenges. To reflect this broad array of conditions and severity levels, and help define the scope of required integration activities and policies, the term 'co-occurring conditions' has been used in some key documents and knowledge exchange activities.[3] In this chapter we use the terms 'mental health–substance use disorders' and 'mental health–substance use conditions' interchangeably.

To go beyond a strictly diagnostic (i.e. categorical) approach to defining co-occurring disorders, Canadian investigators have recently proposed that our definitions and corresponding service planning be grounded in a multidimensional view of problem severity. Problem severity, in this context, consists of three dimensions: acuity, chronicity and complexity.[4]

➤ **Acuity** refers *to short duration and/or urgent risks or adverse consequences* (e.g. physical accident or criminal charges) that are associated with the index problem (e.g. mental health, substance use).
➤ **Chronicity** refers to the development or worsening of *long duration or enduring* conditions (e.g. major depression, hepatitis C).
➤ **Complexity** refers to the *degree of co-occurrence of the index problems and/or the existence of health and social factors* (e.g. chronic pain, homelessness) that complicate the process of addressing the index problem.

Building upon this multidimensional framework of problem severity, the overall 'treatment system' must respond effectively and efficiently to the full spectrum of acute, chronic and often complex needs. This perspective on the 'who' part of the integration issue is not unlike what has been advocated in the management of other health problems such as cardiovascular disease, cancer and diabetes (i.e. so-called chronic care models[5-7]) since essentially it is grounded in a population health framework. Figure 12.1 illustrates the distribution of problem severity for mental health, substance use and mental health–substance use conditions within the general population.

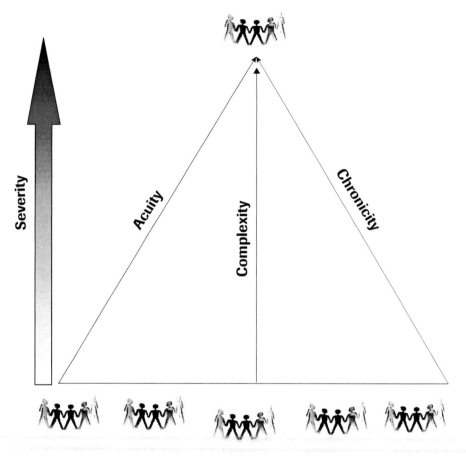

FIGURE 12.1 Target populations for integration efforts by problem severity

A system design framework that supports better integration

Using the population health pyramid as a frame of reference for describing the target population for integration efforts leads one quite naturally to a 'tiered framework' of health systems, in this case the broad mental health and substance use system. Such frameworks now underpin planning efforts in Canada,[8,9] the UK,[10] and parts of Europe.[11]

One such tiered framework has been recommended as the basis of an integrated service delivery system for mental health, substance use and co-occurring conditions in Ontario, Canada.[9] The framework (*see* Figure 12.2) aligns the *functions* of a comprehensive, multi-sectoral system in five tiers that correspond to the acuity, chronicity and complexity of people's needs.

In the context of the five tiers, a **function** refers to a higher-order grouping of like services or interventions aimed at achieving similar outcomes. A 'function' may be:

≫ a component along the continuum of care (e.g. outpatient or residential treatment)

≫ a broad class of interventions (e.g. screening, self-management, pharmacotherapy)

≫ a type of risk management/reduction (e.g. psychosocial crisis intervention, needle exchange)

≫ a population-based initiative (e.g. health promotion)

≫ or any of a variety of types of general counselling and support (e.g. continuing care, case management, peer support).

A function is distinct from a type of program or service (e.g. a primary care setting) and there may well be a range of functions provided in a given service delivery setting. See the recent Canadian report for a complete description and examples of functions and tiers.[9]

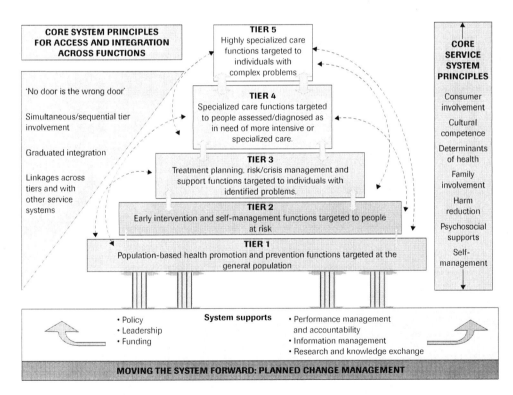

FIGURE 12.2 Tiered framework for designing integrated mental health and substance use systems (Reprinted with the kind permission of the Centre for Addiction and Mental Health, Canada.)

The tiers reflect an increasing degree of specialisation with respect to the nature of the function provided and the expected competency of the service provider to address mental health, substance use and mental health–substance use conditions. This increased degree of specialisation corresponds to increased problem severity (as described in Figure 12.1), such that the higher the tier, the fewer the number of people in need of the service. This also implies a lower requirement to have the functions in the top tiers physically located geographically in all jurisdictions.

Of critical importance to the tiered framework is the fact that individuals and their families can enter this comprehensive service and support system at multiple points (i.e. the concept of 'any door is the right door') and, upon entry, should be linked to other functions within or across tiers according to their needs.[8,10] Thus, the system must be *operationalised* in such a way as to facilitate **transitions** within and across the tiered functions as dictated by the individual's needs – no part of the system 'owns the person'; they are 'individuals' of the entire system. The concept of 'graduated integration' is also critical here, whereby the need for, and intensity of, specific integration strategies are considered in relation to the *severity of the specific sub-population of concern.*

In sum, the population health pyramid helps us get a fix on the overall population that should ostensibly benefit from better integrated mental health and substance use services and systems. Using this population health perspective leads to a broad tiered framework that requires one to step outside of the traditional, and limiting, view of the *specialised* mental health and substance use sectors. In turn, it then forces consideration and concrete planning of graduated integration strategies that will ensure effective transitions within and across tiers (essentially excellent continuity of care), and optimal outcomes.

Distinguishing between service- and system-level integration

Literature that has focused on mental health–substance use disorders has drawn the distinction between **service-level** and **system-level** integration in an attempt to bring more clarity to the discussion of key concepts, and to support research and knowledge translation concerning various integration strategies.[1,12] The Canadian best practices report on co-occurring disorders[2] also clearly articulated that integration did not necessarily mean administrative merger of mental health and substance use services, but rather that organisations, and the services they offer, can work together to ensure an integrated treatment experience for people seeking help.

Service-level integration

The seminal reviews by Drake and colleagues on the need for service integration for people with mental health–substance use disorders drew the important distinction between integrated treatment and either sequential or parallel treatment.[13–15] *Sequential (serial) treatment* was defined as treatment that deals with one disorder first, and in isolation, followed by interventions for the second disorder; often using differing treatment approaches (e.g. the medical model for mental disorders, the recovery model for substance use disorders). *Parallel treatment* was defined as treatment that addresses both problems at the same time, but treatments are in isolation of each other, and applying different approaches. In contrast *service integration* was viewed at the *clinical interface* with the individual, whereby they receive interventions that share common ground in terms of programme philosophy; take a long-term approach; and rely on the same team or teams to give consistent explanations and proposed treatment and support strategies.

Integrated clinical care and psychosocial support can also be delivered by well-coordinated, collaborative arrangements *across two or more service providers and not only in co-located programmes*. Recent publications like the 2007 CSAT Co-occurring Centre of Excellence (COCE) Technical Overview Paper Series define integrated services in a way that includes *both* single site and multi-site options among a range of integration configurations.[16]

We adopt the following definition of service-level integration: '*Integrated clinical care and psychosocial support delivered either by co-located teams or well-coordinated, collaborative arrangements across two or more service providers that ensure access to services and supports and effective continuity of care*.'[9]

System-level integration

System-level integration places more emphasis on factors that are required to ensure an individual's access to, and engagement with, a continuum of services appropriate to their needs, such as policy, resource allocation, governance, leadership and performance monitoring. The tiered framework in Figure 12.2 aims to reflect this emphasis by locating 'system supports' as foundational to effective delivery of the functions embedded in the five tiers.

A review distinguished between system- and programme/service-level approaches to integration of health services generally.[17] This review identified several system-level conceptual approaches, ranging from a focus on the key dimensions of a system to an emphasis on change management. They identified 10 'universal core' principles which were frequently and consistently presented in the reviewed literature:

1 Comprehensive services across a continuum of care
2 Clear person focus
3 Geographic coverage and rostering
4 Standardised care delivery (e.g. guidelines and pathways) through inter-professional teams
5 Well-developed performance monitoring systems including indicators
6 Appropriate information systems to track utilisation and outcomes
7 Strong leadership, shared vision and congruent organisational culture
8 Physician integration
9 Strong, focused governance structure
10 Complementary approaches to funding (e.g. population-based funding).

While similar principles are identified in a review by the Change Foundation[18] authors point out that there is little evidence to demonstrate which principles, if any, are more relevant, or if a certain combination leads to more successful integration.[17] We adopt the following definition of system-level integration:

> Structures and processes that provide the infrastructure for the organization and delivery of integrated clinical and psychosocial services and supports for people with mental health, substance use, problem gambling and co-occurring conditions and their families. These include key system

level functions that government and/or regional health authorities need to address in order to support integrated services. This includes supports such as policy, leadership, funding, performance measurement and accountability, information management, human resource management, and research and knowledge exchange.[9]

MAKING THE CASE FOR BETTER INTEGRATION

Building the case for integration of mental health and substance use services and systems for people experiencing mental health–substance use disorders has evolved through three overlapping but distinctive stages:[19]

➤ The *discovery* stage (i.e. what are the problems or key issues?).
➤ The *significance* stage (i.e. how important are they?).
➤ The *programme/policy solutions* stage (what are potential clinical and system strategies to improve and support integration activities, and do these strategies yield positive outcomes?).

The primary literature in each stage emanated originally from the United States, which in turn stimulated similar work in other countries, especially Canada, the UK, Australia and New Zealand, and together has contributed substantively to the evidence base in the area. That said, it is critical that jurisdictions seek to replicate the core findings on mental health–substance use disorders within their own context. This is because unique historical, social and cultural issues are likely to be important at each stage of research and development in a given jurisdiction, and have implications for planning concrete integration strategies. This is especially true for understanding the basic epidemiology of mental and substance use disorders, including mental health–substance use disorders, and factors challenging the delivery of comprehensive and effective services.

Stage one: the literature on 'discovery'

During the discovery stage, the emphasis in the research is on understanding the degree of overlap among mental health and substance use disorders. The call for more integrated services and systems was stimulated in large part by community psychiatric epidemiological studies in the United States demonstrating high overlap in the general population. The Epidemiologic Catchment Area (ECA) Survey,[20] initially administered between 1980 and 1984, found that individuals with a mental illness were at substantially increased odds of also experiencing a substance use disorder in their lifetime, and vice versa. This was particularly true for specific disorders where the likelihood of having a substance use disorder was substantially higher than for the general population – four times for individuals with schizophrenia and five times for those with bipolar disorder. Subsequent prevalence studies reported rates of overlap typically in the 20%–40% range for alcohol use disorders and 30%–50% for drug use disorders.[21] The findings, however, depended considerably on the country, the measures, the time period under study (e.g. lifetime versus 12-month estimates), and other methodological issues.[22]

Community studies also confirmed that the degree of overlap is even higher among adolescents.[23] Data from good quality population-based longitudinal studies of children and adolescents are particularly relevant as they show many common risk factors for substance use and mental disorders, as well as the persistence of such disorders from adolescence to adulthood.[24] Importantly, the vast majority of substance use disorders in adolescence and young adulthood are predated by mental health problems in childhood or adolescence (*see* Chapters 6 and 7).[25-28] These findings have unrecognised potential for prevention.

It is important to note that recent survey estimates suggest the degree of overlap is much less than previously reported, at least for adults in the general population. In 2004, the National Epidemiologic Survey on Alcohol and Related Conditions (NESARC) found about 20% of all persons in the general population with a current substance use disorder also had at least one current independent mood disorder; and 18% had at least one current independent anxiety disorder. Similarly, about 20% of those with at least one current independent *mood* disorder had a co-occurring substance use disorder, and 15% of those with at least one 12-month independent *anxiety* disorder had a substance use disorder.[29] One possible factor underlying the lower rates of mental health–substance use disorders compared to the landmark National Comorbidity Study (NCS) and Epidemiological Catchment Area (ECA) studies was the use of a more stringent and accurate protocol for defining substance use disorders according to DSM-IV. Published Canadian data[30] also showed rates of overlap consistent with the most recent US data from the NESARC survey, and in the 15%–20% range depending on the denominator employed. Thus, the recent data, including data published for co-occurring substance use and personality disorders, are quite consistent in showing that the majority of people *in the general population* with mental and substance use disorders do *not* have mental health–substance use disorders.

A large literature also blossomed over this period (roughly between 1990 and 2004) on the frequency and presentation of mental health–substance use disorders in clinical settings, including both substance use and mental health services. Higher rates of mental health–substance use disorders were commonly found among individuals attending specialised substance use services (typically in the 60%–70% range) compared to mental health services (typically within 20%–50%).[19] However, two studies of comprehensive mental health systems (as opposed to studies in individual treatment settings) show rates of overlap close to 15%–50%.[31,32] This is far below what is typically reported in equally comprehensive studies of substance use services.[33] However, what Rush and Koegl did observe in the mental health system were much higher rates of overlap among certain sub-populations, in particular, young males with personality disorders.[32]

Researchers have also looked beyond mental health and substance use services specifically, and examined the degree of overlap in substance use and mental disorders in other settings such as emergency departments,[34] and correctional facilities.[35] In particular, the high degree of overlap in correctional settings (in the 90% range) has drawn considerable attention (*see* Chapter 14).

In summary, for substance use services, mental health–substance use disorders are clearly the rule rather than the exception. This may be due in part to the neurotoxic effects of substance use; that is, heavy substance use manifestations of sub-clinical mental illness can increase in severity and duration and reach clinical thresholds. In contrast, among people seeking treatment and support from mental health services, mental health–substance use disorders are, in fact, the exception rather than the rule, unless one is focused on specific *sub-populations* and unique types of services. These differences in the context and population in which mental health–substance use disorders are being examined have important implications for service planning and delivery, particularly as they relate to the motivations and challenges for integration across the two service systems.

Stage two: the literature on 'significance'

During the late 1970s and early 1980s, researchers in the United States reported on the poorer community adjustment and higher rates of re-admission to hospital among young people with severe mental illnesses, such as schizophrenia, and who also 'abused' alcohol and other drugs.[36–38] Later research began to emerge demonstrating that mental health–substance use disorders were associated with poorer clinical and social outcomes than those associated with either disorder in isolation. Examples include higher rates of relapse and rehospitalisation,[39,40] depression and suicidality,[41] violence,[42] incarceration,[35] homelessness,[43,44] family dysfunction,[45] and HIV and hepatitis C infection.[46]

Research emanating from the substance use field yielded similar concerns regarding co-occurring mental illness, particularly as it relates to treatment outcomes.[47–51] The negative impact of psychiatric comorbidity on substance use treatment outcomes has since been replicated many times.[52–54] Flynn and Brown[19] have argued that an important finding in these outcome studies has been given much too little attention – namely, that the impact of the comorbidity, and the benefits of various integrated treatment options, are highly dependent on the *severity* of the mental disorder and associated functioning.

The early population surveys noted above consistently indicated that a significant proportion of people with either a mental or substance use disorder (or both) does not seek services,[21,55,56] a finding exacerbated among adolescents.[24] Results from a more recent household survey in the US reported that 72% of those with co-occurring disorders had not received any specialty mental health or substance use services and only 8% had received both.[57] Harris and Edlund[58] reported that 65% of individuals with a co-occurring disorder did not receive any help, and that this also depends on problem severity (with the more severe being more likely to receive some treatment).

Although the level of unmet need is extremely high, individuals experiencing mental health–substance use disorders are, in fact, more likely to seek care than those with mental or substance use disorders alone,[20,21,55,59–61] although the data are not consistent in this regard for adolescents experiencing mental health–substance use disorders.[24] This higher propensity for help seeking was another fundamental driving force behind the call for improved integration emanating from the early epidemiological surveys on mental health–substance use disorders.

Importantly, the survey data also showed that in spite of this tendency for help seeking, and the high prevalence rates and poor clinical and social outcomes for this group, the vast majority of individuals experiencing mental health–substance use disorder were not receiving adequate care.[1,57] The review by Flynn and Brown[19] reported that only a minority of substance use services provided programmes for people experiencing mental health–substance use disorders. For adolescents with co-occurring disorders, even among those with identified disorders, only a minority received treatment.[62] Several studies also clearly suggest that, given a mental health–substance use disorder, the chances of receiving help in a substance use service for a mental health problem are substantially higher than receiving help for a substance use problem in a mental health service.[19] These findings are especially troubling for some sub-populations given that problems with substance abuse tend to be chronic for individuals with a severe mental illness,[13] and this chronicity contributes to multiple relapses of psychotic symptoms, heavy substance use, and multiple treatment admissions. One study reported that individuals experiencing mental health–substance use disorder reported the lowest satisfaction with care and were four to seven times more likely to report unmet need compared to those with either a substance use or mental disorder alone.[61]

Early reviews of mental health and substance use systems in the United States showed that when individuals experiencing mental health–substance use disorder did seek help, they were confronted with the realities of separate mental health and substance use systems, including policy, financing and regulatory barriers, poor information flow, various restrictions on admission, and disparate messages and philosophy regarding treatment and recovery.[63] Other systems-level studies also reinforced the importance of attitudinal factors, social stigma, professional 'turfism' and lack of resources as presenting barriers to optimal care.[64–70] If able to access required services at all, the typical result was a failure to engage, motivate and retain people in treatment.[1,13,14]

There is strong evidence that the 'double trouble' of mental health–substance use disorders is reflected in the costs of providing treatment and support, and that these costs are distributed in many parts of the health and social service systems. For example, one study found that among individuals with schizophrenia receiving services in a community mental health centre, those who were currently misusing substances were more likely to use institutional services of all kinds, including correctional services, substance abuse-related hospitalisation, and emergency services, as compared to those who had substance use problems in the past and those with no history of substance use problems.[71] The average annual service costs for the three groups varied accordingly, with the highest costs going to those currently experiencing substance use problems. Research synthesised in a recent review of mental health–substance use disorders and adolescence illustrates the exacerbated costs of such comorbidity at a young age.[24,71]

Stage three: the literature on 'programme/policy solutions'
Service-level integration
Broadly speaking, improved 'integration' at the service level is touted as the solution to challenges that have been experienced by people with co-occurring disorders with sequential or parallel treatment and support. The most influential literature reviews concerning integrated treatment were published by Drake and colleagues in 1998,[13] again in 2004[14] and, more recently, in 2008.[15] The first two reviews pointed towards the value of integrated treatment models of service delivery that espoused

key principles including stage-wise treatment; engagement and motivational counselling interventions; active treatment (e.g. counselling to promote adherence, behavioural skills training); relapse prevention, long-term retention, and comprehensive services such as housing and educational and health-related supports, and interventions for treating non-responders.

Interestingly, in the 2008 review by this same group, integration was taken more as a given rather than a central aspect of the research question. That is, the primary focus of the research synthesis was on the evidence for specific psychosocial interventions that could be included in an integrated model (e.g. individual or group counselling, family intervention, residential or outpatient treatment, contingency management and legal interventions such as jail diversion or other forms of mandated treatment or monitoring). The evidence was said to be strongest for group counselling, contingency management and long-term residential treatment. However, a more ecological approach to the delivery and evaluation of services was also advanced, for example, taking into account the environmental context in which the person lives, and in which the service itself is located. A tailored approach was recommended with different types of interventions seen as more appropriate for some types of sub-groups and settings (e.g. emphasising engagement strategies for people who are homeless). A *sequenced* approach was also recommended in some situations, borrowing the concept of stepped-care from the substance use field[72-74] and other branches of psychological therapy.[75] In a stepped-care model, less intensive and expensive interventions are tried first, then, contingent on the initial response to the first level of care, are followed by more extensive and expensive interventions. Improved use of electronic decision-support systems was also recommended. As mentioned earlier, these key ingredients were to be delivered in the context of an integrated, co-located service.

While the emphasis in the reviews by Drake and colleagues, and many other experts, has been on integrated clinical teams, the definition of service-level integration also includes well-coordinated, collaborative arrangements across two or more service providers. There has, however, been limited research addressing the question of comparative effectiveness of single-site versus collaborative-care models. Indeed, only relatively recently was a comparison of these two approaches a specific focus of research enquiry.[76] The results showed that the two options did *not* differ in terms of access to services, or other outcomes.

Recent literature reviews and formal meta-analyses of the integration literature, again at the services level, have been conducted and conclude with a more cautionary message as to the need for integration.[77,78] One study selected the best 10 studies, from a methodological point of view, of integrated versus non-integrated treatment.[77] All were randomised controlled trials – one comparing integrated and parallel treatment options; seven comparing integrated and standard treatment in mental health services; and two comparing integrated and standard treatment in substance use services. Using improvement in symptoms as the outcome criteria, little evidence was found favouring the integrated treatment options. Modest to strong evidence, however, was found for improvements in treatment engagement/compliance and outcomes related to social adjustment.

The most recent research synthesis focused on the effectiveness of psychosocial treatment for people with both severe and persistent mental illness and substance use problems.[78] However, rather than starting from a position that all these interventions would best be delivered in an integrated context, they considered integrated treatment as one of several intervention models to be contrasted with standard care. The other treatment options were non-integrated treatment, cognitive behavioural therapy, motivational interviewing, and life skills training. Results showed that in order to reduce substance use or improve mental health status, there was no compelling evidence to support any one psychosocial intervention over another, including integrated treatment.

What all the experts reviewing the literature in this area do agree upon is that, although the quality of research in the area is improving, the *synthesis* of valid literature on service integration remains severely challenged by a host of issues such as varying outcome measures, settings and samples. Thus, the informed reader needs to be aware that, at the service level, the value of integrated services is not clear-cut and much more work needs to be done, particularly with sub-groups based on clinical features and problem severity.

A review[9] cited the following list of evidence-informed service integration mechanisms for mental health and substance use services:

- service information that is centralised and accessible to providers and the general public
- centralised intake and assessment, or at least a coordinated intake and assessment process with common, standardised tools and processes
- integrated, single records or protocols for sharing information
- shared best practice clinical guidelines/protocols
- interagency service delivery teams with formal contracts/agreements
- co-location of services/programmes
- case management models (Intensive Case Management, Assertive Community Treatment)
- boundary spanning positions (other case managers, System Navigators)
- protocols for sharing individuals with multiple, complex needs.

As clearly articulated in the tiered framework (Figure 12.2), the conceptual boundaries of 'integration' do not begin or end at the doors of the mental health and substance use service sectors, but should be inclusive of multiple sectors spanning, for example, primary care, social assistance, education, housing, justice/corrections. Indeed, strong arguments can be made that, rather than focus exclusively on the integration of mental health and substance use services, a more appropriate use of expertise and resources would be devoted to better integrating mental health and substance use services and systems *and* health services generally, in particular primary care.[12]

Over the last 10 years or so, shared or collaborative mental healthcare has moved from being a 'fringe' area of practice to one that is increasingly seen as an integral part of the mental healthcare delivery system.[79] The literature on shared/collaborative substance use services and support is not as well developed, although there are increasing references for the need to have effective linkages between these providers and systems.[12] There is also a variety of models for delivering primary care services, varying in potential for integrating mental health and substance services (e.g. Family Health Teams [FHTs], Community Health Centres, [CHCs] and Nurse Practitioner-led Clinics).

System-level integration

There are a wide range of system-level strategies and infrastructure that can be implemented in support of improved integration at the service level. Given this wide range, and since administrators and planners often move quickly to structural solutions, it is important to separate governance/administrative integration (i.e. structural merger) and other kinds of activities and strategies, such as joint planning and e-health solutions to information exchange.

The purpose of different system-level integration activities and strategies also varies. Some system integration processes are concerned with securing or enhancing an adequate resource base, often a critically important, but covert, goal of integration. Other activities and supports aim for more cost-efficient administrative operations such as human resources, information technology, procurement and the like.

Some examples of system-level supports and strategies include formal or continuing education and credentialing; mental health and substance use policy for accessing or financing services; joint planning; e-health initiatives that support and safeguard the transfer of information; and performance indicators and other types of quality improvement processes.

Importantly, the onus of responsibility lies with system-level planners and administrators to:

1 Estimate the cost of proposed system-level supports and strategies.
2 Articulate how proposed initiatives will directly or indirectly impact operations and person/family-centred outcomes.
3 Identify the mechanism that will be used to track and report on success in achieving predetermined goals.

A logic model that 'connects the dots' back to individual and family-related outcomes is an essential part of system-level planning and evaluation (*see* Durbin, Goering, Streiner, *et al.* for a template of such a system-level logic model[80]).

Although ideas and assumptions abound for system-level integration, there is a dearth of research and evaluation data that point to best practice evidence. There is an abundance of proposed strategies and system planning tools to deal with challenges to better integration and help guide the assessment and prioritisation of various types of system supports.[81,82] However, most of the literature on the evaluation of integration approaches has been at the service level.[83–86] Even in the exhaustive literature reviews undertaken by Drake and colleagues, no evidence is brought forward that speaks directly to either the added value of system-level integration, or the necessary/sufficient features at the system level that are required to support integration at the service level.

One study conducted a review of the five best-designed and resourced projects focused on the system level,[80] including one project concerned with the structural integration of mental health and substance use services and services.[87,88] They found no evidence of impact on 'client-level' outcomes (e.g. symptom reduction, quality of life, housing or work status), but acknowledged the many challenges in establishing the link from the system level to such outcomes.

That said, the major contribution of the paper[80] was that system-level integration strategies were positively and consistently related to improved *intermediate continuity-of-care outcomes.* In other words, when the outcomes examined were more proximally connected to the integration supports and strategies, the evidence was much stronger than observed for the more distal health outcomes per se. When they went on to examine the data for critical features that might help explain the associations, they concluded that system-level integration was more effective when characterised by stronger management arrangements, fewer service sectors involved and system-wide implementation of intensive case management and centralised access to services. Thus, there is some evidence supporting systems-level integration if it is targeted, relatively circumscribed and person-focused on access and navigation.

In the United States, findings from research syntheses and major epidemiological surveys have recently stimulated a proliferation of infrastructure and capacity-building initiatives *aimed specifically at improving and sustaining integration activities and processes.*[89,90] Many of these initiatives have been conducted under the national leadership of the Center for Substance Abuse Treatment, SAMHSA. The SAMHSA contributions have included its Report to Congress (Substance Abuse and Mental Health Services Administration, 2002); the Co-occurring State Incentive Grant (COSIG) programme (which supports states in their infrastructure capacity-building efforts); the Co-occurring Center for Excellence (COCE) which disseminates epidemiological data and evidence-based practices; the National Evidence-based Practices Project; the National Registry of Effective Programs,[91] and the widely used Treatment Improvement Protocols (two of which have focused on co-occurring disorders). Changes in infrastructure have also been supported through the National Policy Academy on Co-occurring Substance Abuse and Mental Disorders which brings together key leaders to effect cross-agency collaboration and systems change (in the mental health system, the Federal Mental Health Action Agenda provides a similar support function). Critical to the present discussion on the topic of integration is the fact that this impressive slate of activities supported by SAMHSA and its collaborators has gone well beyond best practice syntheses per se to focus on the development, implementation and evaluation of specific system-level *supports* aimed at addressing barriers that have challenged integration of services and systems for people with co-occurring disorders.

The fact that such supports for integration activities have been strategically implemented in the US acknowledges the reality that system-level (or service-level) integration does not happen simply because someone says it is important, particularly for the two 'silos' separated by deep historical and cultural barriers.

MAKING INTEGRATION HAPPEN

Though the substance use and mental health systems have many things in common there are major differences with respect to such things as policies, approaches to service delivery, staff credentialing and funding. Consequently, there are long-standing barriers to providing integrated services, which need to be understood when planning for system-level (or service-level) changes.[82] These barriers can be categorised at both the system and service levels.

Barriers to better integration

Table 12.1 synthesises a substantive body of literature on the barriers to the integration of mental health and substance use services and systems and draws heavily from reviews.[1,2,11,12,17,92] Some of these reviews provide complementary summaries of strengths and commonalities that can facilitate better integration, synthesised in Box 12.1.

TABLE 12.1 Challenges and barriers that hinder better integration

Service level	System level
Lack of identification of mental health–substance use disorders and no shared screening and assessment tools.	Separate funding allocations, planning structures and governance mechanisms. There is also a lack of long-term planning.
Discriminatory admission policies.	Perceptions of professional inequality and status differences as well as different professional certification requirements.
Different models of service delivery, including medical versus non-medical orientation, use of medication and lack of acceptance of harm-reduction approach. Lack of a common language.	Lack of a full continuum of mental health and substance use services within each sector. Services in both systems are in 'survival mode' and lack resources to serve all those requiring treatment.
No locus of responsibility for care.	Fragmented services for people with co-occurring disorders, particularly those who are homeless or in other ways marginalised.
Individual and families not well informed about mental health–substance use disorders.	Different histories/perceptions of consumer involvement.
Complexity of individuals' problems and lack of support, expertise and clinical supervision.	Individuals experiencing mental health–substance use disorders experience greater stigma.
Resistance to change at professional, team and organisation levels.	Lack of leadership, political will and/or public support.
Difficulties with professional boundaries and responsibilities as well as a reluctance to 'give away' skills.	Lack of resources, including information technology, to support system integration.
Mental health and substance use symptoms interfere with treatment.	Professional training does not include mental health–substance use disorders.

BOX 12.1 Strengths and commonalities that can facilitate better integration at both the service and system levels

- The use of the 'continuum of care' approach to system planning and the need for individualised treatment and support within that continuum.
- The importance of a coordinated network of services in the community that includes specialised services, as well as other services required on a referral basis.
- The need for improved integration with the larger health system and, in particular, with primary care. Viewing primary care as the 'front line' for both mental health and substance use issues; similar protocols and models have been developed for mental health and primary care and substance use and primary care, including screening and brief intervention.
- The importance of self-help resources and family supports.
- The shared challenges of stigma and discrimination – for those seeking care, for their families and friends, and for their service providers.
- The common ground offered by chronic care models of health services and a focus on long-term support and recovery when needed.
- Many common issues related to specific populations (e.g. culturally appropriate treatment and support, special needs of new immigrant populations, such as refugees, and geographically dispersed and isolated populations).
- Issues related to professional competencies, supply and retention are shared between the mental health and substance use sectors.

Clearly, the barriers to better integration operate at multiple levels and require careful planning and implementation in order to address them effectively and in a sustained way. A strengths-based approach is also required in order to capitalise on the many areas of commonality across the two historically siloed sectors.

Broadly speaking, integration activities and processes will also be more effective when guided by theoretical or conceptual models of change management – whether it be at the service (i.e. individual, team, organisation) or the system level. There is a plethora of models to help guide better integration; indeed, so many models are of potential value that it is beyond the scope of this chapter to review them in detail. Reviews of change management are provided within the context of the healthcare system and health service organisations,[93-97] while others have focused on large organisational mergers.[98] Examples of specific approaches to planned change include organisational learning[99] and total quality management[100] or similar frameworks for quality improvement,[101] with some authors arguing for a multilevel approach.[102] Other literature of high relevance includes that concerning diffusion of innovation theory,[103] stages of change,[97] partnerships,[104] vertical versus horizontal integration,[105,106] continuum models of collaboration[107] and continuity-of-care.[80,108]

Notwithstanding the universal call for more research on the effective ingredients of planned change, several lessons for the integration of mental health and substance use services and systems have been drawn from this large body of literature.[9,12,82] The following is a brief synthesis of key factors drawn from these reviews.

➤ **Shared vision**: Ensure that there is a clear, accessible and shared vision, supported by common values, which informs all aspects of organisational and network activities, policies and planning.

➤ **Culture**: Strive to foster an organisational culture that is committed to learning and experimentation that is consistent with the shared vision while still embracing diversity.

➤ **Leadership**: Recognise as a primary responsibility of executive leaders the need to consistently champion the new shared vision, support a developing organisational culture and actively seek out and foster leaders at all levels.

➤ **Social capital**: Recognise the potential of an organisation's social capital – in particular teams – to shape and impact change. Invest, through training, support and development, individuals and teams who share the organisation's vision of change. Be sure to recognise people seeking services as a key component of this social capital.

➤ **Change process**: Devote sufficient resources, both financial and human, to support all stages of the change process – from planning to implementation to performance monitoring – always with a focus on engagement of all members and at all levels.

➤ **Communication**: Support open, regular, two-way communication that facilitates understanding of the need for change, problem-solving to work through change, and feedback to maintain and enhance change.

SYSTEMS THEORY AND INTER-ORGANISATIONAL NETWORK ANALYSIS

In addition to the large body of literature referred to earlier on conceptual models and theories related to change and change management, two additional areas of theory and methodology have been recently identified for advancing integration of mental health and substance use services and systems.[12]

1 **Systems theory** and, specifically, emergence theory and the closely related concept of complex adaptive systems.

2 **Inter-organisational** network analysis.

Systems theory and complex adaptive systems

One of the major challenges in adopting a systems approach to the study of the integration of mental health and substance use services and systems is the 'mind trap' of the traditional view of a 'system'.[109] This view holds that a 'system' is defined as a set of interconnected parts working towards a common purpose (or purposes); for example, how different clinicians and providers work together to achieve positive outcomes. More recent thinking in systems theory goes well beyond this traditional focus on relationships, and the linearity and orderliness embodied within them.[110] True 'systems thinking' acknowledges that many situations, including those involving inter-organisational relationships, are better described as 'emergent', 'unordered' or 'chaotic'. The theoretical lens through which to examine and understand these situations is variously known as 'emergence theory', 'open-systems theory', 'dynamic systems theory' or 'complexity theory'. Complex adaptive systems also embody many of these key concepts.[111]

'Emergence' is considered to be a property of all living systems and is closely tied to the idea that networks form in order to adapt to changing circumstances. Thus, *networks* of individuals and organisations, united behind a common goal, are seen as the primary mechanism of all change processes.[112] Importantly, however, emergence theory goes several steps beyond the description of relationships within a network (e.g. network maps and network roles) to aim for an understanding of the *dynamics* underlying the network (e.g. why they form; why and how leadership evolved; what keeps members connected).

With respect to the integration of mental health and substance use, emergence theory teaches us that real and sustainable change is built from the bottom up among interested individuals, groups and communities rather than through top-down administrative directives. One does not wave a magic wand and just say, 'OK, thou shalt be integrated!' Integration, from an emergence perspective, can be envisioned and nurtured but the outcome cannot be predetermined, and is highly *situation-dependent*. These factors have important implications for both planning and evaluating integration activities and strategies at multiple levels – the service or system levels.

Inter-organisational network theory

Network theory is essentially a theory about the number and degree of connections between various players or actors and the nature of these connections – between a few individuals, departments/units, organisations or larger systems. Generally, networks refer to either naturally or artificially developed relationships among organisations that operate as '*mechanisms for communication, cooperation, and collective problem solving*'.[113] The nature of these relationships depends on a variety of antecedents including, at the interpersonal level, actor similarity, personality, proximity, organisational structure, and environmental factors; at the inter-unit level, interpersonal ties, functional ties, organisational processes and control mechanisms; and at the inter-organisational level, motives, learning, trust, norms and monitoring, and equity and context.[114] Given the potential for the virtually endless combinations and degrees of influences on a network, it soon becomes readily apparent that networks of even modest proportions can be very complex.

Early applications of organisational network analysis focused on mental health services[115] and played a major role in the evaluation of important mental health-related programmes such as the ACCESS project for homelessness in the US.[116] A synthesis of work on the effectiveness of mental health systems identified, for example, that:[117]

➤ Other things being equal, network effectiveness will be enhanced under conditions of general system stability, although stability alone is not a sufficient condition for effectiveness.

➤ In addition, when a network is embedded in a resource-scarce environment, the potential for network effectiveness is greater.

There is also evidence to support building networks based on 'small world' principles, as opposed to 'big world principles', where '*the best network has local clustering into dense sub-networks, short paths between all actors, and relatively few ties*'.[113] Indeed, Provan and Millward[117] present research supporting this claim, suggesting that outcomes are more influenced by linkages between *cliques* (i.e. linkages between sub-groups, members of which share common interests in a client group[118]), than by linkages between all the agencies in a service network or system that are more removed from direct person-centred services (e.g. signing agreements on joint programme delivery). They illustrated, for example, that within a larger network of organisations that was focused broadly on chronic disease management and prevention, the interrelationships among smaller 'cliques' of organisations were correlated with positive health and quality of life outcomes at the individual level. Analysis of the interrelationships among members of the larger network revealed no such pattern. There are important lessons to be drawn here for the integration of mental health and substance use services and systems, and the evaluation of integration strategies.

SUMMARY

There is a notable absence in the literature on both systems theory and inter-organisational network theory as they relate to discussions of mental health and substance use service and systems integration. This is unfortunate from conceptual and methodological points of view as they have much to offer. Systems theory, especially that concerned with 'emergence' and 'complex adaptive systems', teaches us that the process of change inherent in moving towards improved integration at the services and systems-levels is inherently context dependent and most likely non-linear and difficult to control, or centrally micro-manage. Systems and network theory also remind us that effective functional integration and integrative network formation tend to be highly responsive to emergent perceived needs for integration; that development processes are difficult to predict and manage; and that they cannot be effectively mandated.

Both systems-related ideas and network analysis inform us that real and sustainable integration is built from the bottom up or, perhaps more accurately stated, rarely if ever exclusively from the top down. The role of high-level 'big world' systems integration is to support the individually focused and 'small-world' integration processes that begin with professionals and managers. Systems evaluation also requires a thorough and perhaps non-conventional exploration of relationships, perspectives and boundaries,[119] drawing on mixed evaluation methods that go beyond linear logic modelling and causal-based statistical methods. Contextual factors are also critical in interpreting any data on the processes and outcomes of integration.

CONCLUSION: TIERS ARE NOT ENOUGH

The literature reviewed herein has primarily examined the structural conditions required for effective integrated systems and services, with continuity of care and positive health outcomes for the individual being cited as key dependent variables for the measurement of successful integration experience. Outcomes, however, are not only dependent on these structural conditions, but also on factors associated with effective clinical interventions.[120,121] Whatever integrative model is applied, the quality of interactions with the individual at intake and during and after treatment, which may make for either a facilitating or impeding context, must be factored into the mix of effective integrated systems and services.[122-124] What happens behind closed doors with the individual has an essential contribution to the equation of successful outcomes, and it is these microanalytic concerns that take up a better part of the working hours of professionals.

The body of research on treatment effectiveness is substantial and has not been the focus of this chapter. Suffice it to say that a significant portion of these studies has been devoted to the quest for the Holy Grail – that is, the best therapeutic model and the most effective interventions. A clear clinical model provides a needed framework to interpret past, present and future events associated with a disorder. While numerous models and interventions have been shown to be effective for the treatment of substance misuse and mental health problems, and specifically for mental health–substance use disorders, no one intervention has been shown to be superior in all cases and for all individuals.[121,125] To complicate the search, research also demonstrates that models and interventions are not enough – other necessary factors include the need for professionals to believe their approach is effective and to be able to convincingly communicate this belief to the individual.

Another key factor identified in treatment outcome research relates to the professional's capacity to develop an effective working relationship.[124,126] The therapeutic alliance (*see* Book 4, Chapter 2), as many authors describe this working relationship, involves an emotion – a positive feeling between the individual and therapist. This emotion is based in part on the developed consensus between the individual and the therapist on the goals of the intervention, taking into account the individual's expectations. Such a rapport gives hope that recovery is possible, enables engagement and trust in the therapeutic relationship and, outside of this therapeutic context, supports the individual to begin and maintain the process of change. Research has highlighted specific interpersonal skills required by the professional to achieve an effective therapeutic alliance, summarised as the ability to:[127]

➤ express in words what is happening in the clinical process
➤ express emotion
➤ persuade
➤ give hope
➤ express warmth
➤ have empathy
➤ establish an alliance
➤ problem solve.

The tiered framework for designing integrated mental health and substance use systems, presented in Figure 12.2 earlier in this chapter, needs to be revisited, taking into account this clinical context. From Tiers 2 to 5, the manner in which individuals are greeted and treated will determine whether individuals trust that they have knocked on the right door. If the skills needed at Tier 2 differ from those required at Tier 5, one can safely hypothesise that not only shared values and compatible theoretical models but also the use of facilitating interpersonal skills in all tiers are required to increase positive outcomes. Furthermore, the connectedness between the various players and actors that forms the networks foundational to successful integration should also include a common vision regarding the key role of the therapeutic alliance. This is the missing link in the literature and one that can compromise the successful passage of a individual from one programme to another; from one tier to another.[128] Inasmuch as professional support and work towards integrated systems and services – the bottom-up approach – is associated with real and sustainable change, the same is true of professionals whom, at every tier, show they genuinely want to help, are able to communicate that there is hope, and are capable of mobilising the strengths of the person in the service of recovery.

In closing, we trust this chapter has offered 'food for thought' to assist in deliberations on the integration of mental health and substance use services and systems. We hope it proves useful in debriefing on past integration experience and offers concrete support for integration efforts currently under way or being considered. We recognise that our report offers more in terms of the 'whys' and 'whats' of integration and less on the 'hows.' Our essential conclusion is that the 'integration train' has left the station for a wide variety of reasons, and that improved integration offers high potential for more effective services and supports for people experiencing mental health–substance use disorders, as well as for the larger group of persons in the population with mental health or substance use disorders, but which do not co-occur.

An examination of research indicates that many roads lead to Rome and that different integrative trajectories bring forth effective services. Consequently, we suggest that, collectively, we work to avoid the 'integration reflex' and pursue it more thoughtfully and strategically than has been the case in some situations in the past. The strengths and weaknesses of each community or health authority should enter the equation in the process of decision-making as there is no universal solution to the treatment and support of people experiencing mental health–substance use disorders. It is also essential that any integration effort be adequately resourced and supported since many of the changes that are required are in the realm of organisational and systems culture and, therefore, are going to require sustained efforts and ongoing corrective feedback loops to ensure the goals are being met for people needing services and supports. Whatever the choices, interactions between professionals and the individual remain a key component of positive outcomes. In the end, it will be functional integration in service of the individual's needs that make a difference to people's lived experience.

ACKNOWLEDGEMENTS

The authors would like to acknowledge the contributions of several colleagues of Dr Rush at the Health Systems Research and Consulting Unit, Centre for Addiction and Mental Health, in particular, Garth Martin, Dianne Macfarlane, Dale Butterill, Paula Goering and April Furlong – all of whom made significant contributions to the tiered model first presented in a report on the design of an integrated system for mental health and substance use services in Ontario, Canada. We would also like to thank Barry Fogg, formerly with the Manitoba Addictions Foundation, for his contributions to an early report upon which we have drawn extensively. Lastly, our thanks go again to April Furlong for her outstanding support of the preparation of this chapter and previous related work.

REFERENCES

1 Substance Abuse and Mental Health Services Administration. *Report to Congress on the Prevention and Treatment of Co-occurring Substance Abuse Disorders and Mental Disorders.* Washington, DC: Department of Health and Human Services; 2002.

2 Health Canada. *Best Practices: concurrent mental health and substance use disorders.* Ottawa, ON: Health Canada; 2001.

3 Complexities of Co-occurring conditions: harnessing services research to improve care for mental, substance use, and medical/physical disorders. Washington, DC; June 23–25, 2004. Available at: http://archives.drugabuse.gov/meetings/ccc/ (accessed 9 July 2010).

4 Reist D, Brown D. *Exploring Complexity and Severity within a Framework for Understanding Risk Related to Substance Use and Harm.* Unpublished manuscript; December 2008.

5 Wagner EH. Chronic disease management: what will it take to improve care for chronic illness? *Effective Clinical Practice.* 1998; **1**: 2–4.

6 Bodenheimer T, Wagner EH, Grumbach K. Improving primary care for patients with chronic illness: the chronic care model, Part 2. *Journal of the American Medical Association.* 2002; **288**: 1909–14.

7 Wallace PJ. Physician involvement in disease management as part of the CCM. *Health Care Financing Review.* 2005; **27**: 19–31.

8 National Treatment Strategy Working Group. *A Systems Approach to Substance Use in Canada: recommendations for a national treatment strategy.* Ottawa, ON: National Framework for Action to Reduce the Harms Associated with Alcohol and Other Drugs and Substances in Canada; 2008.

9 Health Systems Research and Consulting Unit. *The Design of an Evidence informed, Integrated Mental Health, Substance Use and Problem Gambling Service System for Ontario.* Toronto, ON: Centre for Addiction and Mental Health; 2009.

10 National Treatment Agency for Substance Misuse. *Models of Care for Treatment of Adult Drug Misusers: update 2006.* London: National Treatment Agency for Substance Misuse; 2006.

11 Baldacchino A. Corkery J. *Comorbidity: perspectives across Europe.* London: European Collaborating Centres in Addiction Studies; 2006.

12 Rush B, Fogg B, Nadeau L, *et al. On the Integration of Mental Health and Substance Use Services and Systems.* Ottawa, ON: Canadian Executive Council on Addictions; 2008.

13 Drake RE, Mercer-McFadden C, Mueser KT, *et al.* Review of integrated mental health and substance abuse treatment for patients with dual disorders. *Schizophrenia Bulletin.* 1998; **24**: 589–608.

14 Drake RE, Mueser KT, Brunette MF, *et al.* A review of treatments for people with severe mental illnesses and co-occurring substance use disorders. *Psychiatric Rehabilitation Journal.* 2004; **27**: 360–74.

15 Drake RE, O'Neal EL, Wallach MA. A systematic review of psychosocial research on psychosocial interventions for people with co-occurring severe mental and substance use disorders. *Journal of Substance Abuse Treatment.* 2008; **34**: 123–38.

16 Center for Substance Abuse Treatment. *Co-occurring Centre of Excellence (COCE) Technical Overview Paper Series.* Rockville, MD: Substance Abuse and Mental Health Services Administration, and Center for Mental Health Services; 2007. Available at: www.coce. samhsa.gov/products/overview_papers.aspx (accessed 7 July 2010).

17 Suter E, Oelke ND, Adair CE, *et al. Health Systems Integration. Definitions, processes and impact: a research synthesis.* Calgary, AB: Health Systems and Research Unit, Calgary Health Region; 2007.

18 The Change Foundation. *Integrated Health Care in England: lessons for Ontario.* Toronto, ON: The Change Foundation; 2009.

19 Flynn PM, Brown BS. Co-occurring disorders in substance abuse treatment: issues and prospects. *Journal of Substance Abuse Treatment.* 2008; **34**: 36–47.

20 Regier DA, Farmer ME, Rae DS, *et al.* Comorbidity of mental disorders with alcohol and other drug abuse: results from the Epidemiological Catchment Area (ECA) study. *Journal of the American Medical Association.* 1990; **264**: 2511–18.

21 Kessler RC, Nelson CB, McGonagle KA, *et al.* The epidemiology of co-occurring addictive and mental disorders: implications for prevention and service utilisation. *American Journal of Orthopsychiatry.* 1996; **66**: 17–31.

22 Jané-Llopis E, Matytsina I. Mental health and alcohol, drugs and tobacco: a review of the comorbidity between mental disorders and the use of alcohol, tobacco and illicit drugs. *Drug and Alcohol Review.* 2006; **25**: 515–36.

23 Armstrong TD, Costello EJ. Community studies on adolescent substance use, abuse, or dependence and psychiatric comorbidity. *Journal of Consulting and Clinical Psychology.* 2002; **70**: 1224–39.

24 Adair CE. *Concurrent Substance Use and Mental Disorders in Adolescents: a review of the literature on current science and practice.* Edmonton, AB: Alberta Centre for Child Family and Community Research; 2009.

25 Merikangas KR, Avenevoli S. Implications of genetic epidemiology for the prevention of substance use disorders. *Addictive Behaviors.* 2000; **25**: 807–20.

26 Wise BK, Cuffe SP, Fischer T. Dual diagnosis and successful participation of adolescents in substance abuse treatment. *Journal of Substance Abuse Treatment.* 2001; **21**: 161–5.

27 Costello EJ, Mustillo S, Erkanli A, *et al.* Prevalence and development of psychiatric disorders in childhood and adolescence. *Archives of General Psychiatry.* 2003; **60**: 837–44.

28 Compton SN, Burns BJ, Egger HL, *et al.* Review of the evidence base for treatment of childhood psychopathology: internalizing disorders. *Journal of Consulting and Clinical Psychology.* 2002; **70**: 1240–66.

29 Grant BF, Frederick FS, Dawson A, *et al.* Prevalence and co-occurrence of substance use disorders and independent mood and anxiety disorders. *Archives of General Psychiatry.* 2004; **61**: 807–16.

30 Rush BR, Urbanoski K, Bassani D, *et al.* Prevalence of co-occurring substance use and other mental disorders in the Canadian population. *Canadian Journal of Psychiatry.* 2008; **53**: 800–9.

31 Virgo N, Bennett G, Higgins D, *et al.* The prevalence and characteristics of co-occurring serious mental illness (SMI) and substance abuse or dependence in the patients of Adult Mental Health and Addiction Services in eastern Dorset. *Journal of Mental Health.* 2001; **10**: 175–88.

32 Rush BR, Koegl CJ. Prevalence and profile of people with co-occurring mental and substance use disorders within a comprehensive mental health system. *Canadian Journal of Psychiatry.* 2008; **53**: 810–21.

33 Chan Y, Dennis ML, Funk RR. Prevalence and comorbidity of major internalizing and externalizing problems among adolescents and adults presenting to substance abuse treatment. *Journal of Substance Abuse Treatment.* 2008; **34**: 14–24.

34 McNiel DE, Binder RL. Psychiatric emergency service use and homelessness, mental disorder, and violence. *Psychiatric Services.* 2005; **56**: 699–704.

35 Abram KM, Teplin LA. Co-occurring disorders among mentally ill jail detainees: implications for public policy. *American Psychologist.* 1991; **46**: 1036–45.

36 Caton CLM. The new chronic patient and the system of community care. *Hospital and Community Psychiatry.* 1981; **32**: 475–8.

37 Pepper B, Krishner MC, Ryglewicz H. The young adult chronic patient: overview of a population. *Hospital and Community Psychiatry.* 1981; **32**: 463–9.

38 Bachrach L. The young adult chronic patient: an analytic review of the literature. *Hospital and Community Psychiatry.* 1982; **33**: 189–97.

39 Linszen DH, Dingemans PM, Lenior ME. Cannabis abuse and the course of recent-onset schizophrenia. *Archives of General Psychiatry.* 1994; **51**: 273–9.

40 Swofford CD, Kasckow JW, Scheller-Gilkey G, *et al.* Substance use: a powerful predictor of relapse in schizophrenia. *Schizophrenia Research.* 1996; **20**: 145–51.

41 Bartels SJ, Drake RE, McHugo GJ. Alcohol abuse, depression, and suicidal behavior in schizophrenia. *American Journal of Psychiatry.* 1992; **149**: 394–5.

42 Cuffel BJ, Shumway M, Chouljian TL, *et al.* A longitudinal study of substance use and community violence in schizophrenia. *Journal of Nervous and Mental Disease.* 1994; **182**: 704–8.

43 Drake RE, Osher FC, Noordsy D, *et al.* Diagnosis of alcohol use disorders in schizophrenia. *Schizophrenia Bulletin.* 1990; **16**: 57–67.

44 Caton CLM, Shrout PE, Eagle PF, *et al.* Risk factors for homelessness among schizophrenic men: a case-control study. *American Journal of Public Health.* 1994; **84**: 265–70.

45 Dixon L, McNary S, Lehman A. Substance abuse and family relationships of persons with severe mental illnesses. *American Journal of Psychiatry.* 1995; **152**: 456–8.

46 Rosenberg SD, Goodman LA, Osher FC, *et al.* Prevalence of HIV, hepatitis B, and hepatitis C in people with severe mental illness. *American Journal of Public Health.* 2001; **91**: 31–7.

47 McLellan, AT, Lewis DC, O'Brien CP, *et al.* Drug dependence, a chronic medical illness: implications for treatment, insurance, and outcomes evaluation. *Journal of the American Medical Association.* 2000; **284**: 1689–95.

48 Rounsaville BJ, Dolinsky ZS, Babor TF, *et al.* Psychopathology as a predictor of treatment outcome in alcoholics. *Archives of General Psychiatry.* 1987; **44**: 505–13.

49 Kranzler HR, Del Boca FK, Rounsaville BJ. Comorbid psychiatric diagnosis predicts three-year outcomes in alcoholics: a posttreatment natural history study. *Journal of Studies on Alcohol.* 1996; **57**: 619–26.

50 Lewis CE, Bucholz KK, Spitznagel E. Effects of gender and comorbidity on problem drinking in a community sample. *Alcohol: Clinical and Experimental Research.* 1996; **20**: 466–76.

51 Pettinati HM, Pierce JD, Belden PP, *et al.* The relationship of Axis II personality disorders to other known predictors of addiction treatment outcomes. *American Journal on Addictions.* 1999; **8**: 136–47.

52 McLellan AT, Lewis DC, O'Brien CP, *et al.* Drug dependence, a chronic medical illness: implications for treatment, insurance, and outcomes evaluation. *Journal of the American Medical Association.* 2000; **284**: 1689–95.

53 Mertens JR, Lu YW, Parthasarathy S, *et al.* Medical and psychiatric conditions of alcohol and drug treatment patients in an HMO. *Archives of Internal Medicine.* 2003; **163**: 2511–17.

54 Weisner C, Matzger H. A prospective study of the factors influencing entry to alcohol and drug treatment. Special section. *Journal of Behavioral Health Services & Research.* 2002; **29**: 126–37.

55 Regier D A, Narrow WE, Rae DS, *et al.* The de facto US mental and addictive disorders service system: epidemiologic catchment area prospective 1-year prevalence rates of disorders and services. *Archives of General Psychiatry.* 1993; **50**: 85–94.

56 Kessler RC, McGonagle KA, Zhao S, *et al.* Lifetime and 12-month prevalence of DSM-III-R psychiatric disorders in the United States. *Archives of General Psychiatry.* 1994; **51**: 8–19.

57 Watkins KE, Burnam A, Kung F, *et al*. A national survey of care for persons with co-occurring mental and substance use disorders. *Psychiatric Services*. 2001; **52**: 1062–8.

58 Harris KM, Edlund MJ. Use of mental health care and substance abuse treatment among adults with co-occurring disorders. *Psychiatric Services*. 2005; **56**: 954–9.

59 Wu L-T, Kouzis AC, Leaf PJ. Influence of comorbid alcohol and psychiatric disorders on utilization of mental health services in the National Comorbidity Survey. *American Journal of Psychiatry*. 1990; **156**: 1230–6.

60 Ross HE, Lin E, Cunningham J. Mental health service use: a comparison of treated and untreated individuals with substance use disorders in Ontario. *Canadian Journal of Psychiatry*. 1999; **44**: 570–7.

61 Urbanoski KA, Rush BR, Wild TC, *et al*. Use of mental health care services by Canadians with co-occurring substance dependence and mental disorders. *Psychiatric Services*. 2007; **58**: 962–9.

62 Bukstein OG, Cornelius J, Trunzo AC, *et al*. Clinical predictors of treatment in a population of adolescents with alcohol use disorders. *Addictive Behaviors*. 2005; **30**: 1663–73.

63 Ridgely MS, Osher FC, Goldman HH, *et al. Executive Summary: chronic mentally ill young adults with substance abuse problems. A review of research, treatment, and training issues.* Baltimore, MD: Mental Health Services Research Center, University of Maryland School of Medicine; 1987.

64 Drake RE, Essock SM, Shaner A, *et al*. Implementing dual diagnosis services for clients with severe mental illness. *Psychiatric Services*. 2001; **52**: 469–76.

65 Young NK, Grella CE. Mental health and substance abuse treatment services for dually diagnosed clients: Results of a statewide survey of county administrators. *Journal of Behavioral Health Services & Research*. 1998; **25**: 83–92.

66 Gretta CE, Gil-Rivas V, Cooper L. Perceptions of mental health and substance abuse program administrators and staff on service delivery to persons with co-occurring substance abuse and mental disorders. *Journal of Behavioral Health Services & Research*. 2004; **31**: 38–49.

67 Todd FC, Sellman JD, Robertson PJ. Barriers to optimal care for patients with coexisting substance use and mental health disorders. *Australian and New Zealand Journal of Psychiatry*. 2002; **36**: 792–9.

68 Todd J, Green G, Harrison M, *et al*. Social exclusion in clients with comorbid mental health and substance misuse problems. *Social Psychiatry and Psychiatric Epidemiology*. 2004; **39**: 581–7.

69 Burnam MA, Watkins KE. Substance abuse with mental disorders: Specialized public systems and integrated care. *Health Affairs*. 2006; **25**: 648–58.

70 McGovern MP, Xie H, Segal SR, *et al*. Addiction treatment services and co-occurring disorders: prevalence estimates, treatment practices, and barriers. *Journal of Substance Abuse Treatment*. 2006; **31**: 267–75.

71 Bartels SJ, Teague GB, Drake RE, *et al*. Substance abuse in schizophrenia: service utilization and costs. *Journal of Nervous and Mental Disease*. 1993; **181**: 227–32.

72 Breslin C, Sobell MB, Sobell LC, *et al*. Problem drinkers: evaluation of a stepped care approach. *Journal of Substance Abuse*. 1998; **10**: 217–32.

73 Sobell MB, Sobell LC. Stepped care for alcohol problems: an efficient method for planning and delivering clinical services. In: Tucker JA, Donovan DM, Marlatt JA, editors. *Changing Addictive Behavior: bridging clinical and public health strategies*. New York: Guilford Press; 1999. pp. 331–43.

74 Sobell MB, Sobell LC. Stepped care as a heuristic approach to the treatment of alcohol problems. *Journal of Consulting and Psychology*. 2000; **68**: 573–9.

75 Bower P, Gilbody S. Stepped care in psychological therapies: access, effectiveness and efficiency. Narrative literature review. *British Journal of Psychiatry.* 2005; **186**: 11–17.

76 Rosenheck RA, Resnick SG, Morissey JP. Closing service system gaps for homeless clients with a dual diagnosis: integrated teams and interagency cooperation. *Journal of Mental Health Policy and Economics.* 2003; **6**: 77–87.

77 Donald M, Dower J, Kavanagh D. Integrated versus non-integrated management and care for clients with co-occurring mental health and substance use disorders: a qualitative systematic review of randomised controlled trials. *Social Science & Medicine.* 2005; **60**: 1371–83.

78 Cleary M, Hunt GE, Matheson S, *et al.* Psychosocial treatment programs for people with both severe mental illness and substance misuse. *Schizophrenia Bulletin.* 2008; **34**: 226–8.

79 Kates N, Gagné MA, Whyte JM. Collaborative mental health care in Canada: looking back and looking ahead. *Canadian Journal of Community Mental Health.* 2008; **27**: 1–4.

80 Durbin J, Goering P, Streiner DL, *et al.* Continuity of care: validation of a new self-report measure for individuals using mental health services. *Journal of Behavioral Health Services & Research.* 2004; **31**: 279–96.

81 Zialogic. *Co-occurring Disorders Toolkit.* Available at: www.zialogic.org/Toolkit_1.htm (accessed 7 July 2010).

82 Carver, V. *Strategies for Planning Integrated Systems for People with Concurrent Substance Use and Mental Health Problems.* Toronto, ON: Centre for Addiction and Mental Health; 2004.

83 Siegfried, N. A review of comorbidity: major mental illness and problematic substance use. *Australian and New Zealand Journal of Psychiatry.* 1998; **32**: 707–17.

84 RachBeisel J, Scott J, Dixon L. Co-occurring severe mental illness and substance use disorders: a review of recent research. *Psychiatric Services.* 1999; **50**: 1427–34.

85 Zweben JE. Severely and persistently mentally ill substance abusers: clinical and policy issues. *Journal of Psychoactive Drugs.* 2000; **32**: 383–9.

86 Brunette MF, Mueser KT. Psychosocial interventions for the long-term management of patients with severe mental illness and co-occurring substance use disorder. *Journal of Clinical Psychiatry.* 2006; **67**(Suppl. 7): 10–17.

87 Bickman L. A continuum of care. More is not always better. *The American Psychologist.* 1996; **51**: 689–710.

88 Bickman L, Noser K, Summerfelt WT. Long-term effects of a system of care on children and adolescents. *The Journal of Behavioral Health Services & Research.* 1999; **26**: 185–202.

89 Power K, DeMartino R. Co-occurring disorders and achieving recovery: the substance abuse and mental health services administration perspective. *Biological Psychiatry.* 2004; **56**: 721–2.

90 Clark HW, Power AK, Le Fauve CE, *et al.* Policy and practice implications of epidemiological surveys on co-occurring mental and substance use disorders. *Journal of Substance Abuse Treatment.* 2008; **24**: 3–13.

91 Torrey WC, Drake RE, Dixon L, *et al.* Implementing evidence-based practices for persons with severe mental illnesses. *Psychiatric Services.* 2001; **52**: 45–50.

92 Ridgely MS, Goldman HH, Willenbring M. Barriers to the care of persons with dual diagnosis: organizational and financing issues. *Schizophrenia Bulletin.* 1990; **16**: 123–32.

93 Bamford D, Daniel S. A case study of change management effectiveness within the NHS. *Journal of Change Management.* 2005; **5**: 391–406.

94 By RT. Organizational change management: a critical review. *Journal of Change Management.* 2009; **5**: 369–80.

95 Iles V, Sutherland K. *Managing Change in the NHS. Organizational change: a review for*

health care managers, professionals and researchers. London: National Co-ordinating Centre for NHS Service Delivery and Organization, National Health Service; 2001.

96 Riley B L, Garcia JM, Edwards NC. Organizational change for obesity prevention – perspectives, possibilities and potential pitfalls. In: Kumanvika S, Brownson RC, editors. *Handbook of Obesity Prevention: a resource for health professionals.* New York: Springer; 2007. pp. 239–61.

97 Prochaska JM, Prochaska JO, Levesque DA. A transtheoretical approach to changing organizations. *Administration and Policy in Mental Health.* 2001; **28**: 247–61.

98 Macfarlane D, Butterill D. From principles to practice: the management of post-merger integration. *Healthcare Quarterly.* 1999; **3**: 35–9.

99 Senge PM. *The Fifth Discipline: the art and practice of the learning organization.* New York: Doubleday; 2006.

100 Adair CE, Simpson E, Casebeer AL, *et al.* Performance measurement in healthcare: part II – state of the science findings by stage of the performance measurement process. *Health Care Policy.* 2006; **2**: 56–78.

101 Glickman SW, Baggett KA, Kurbert CG, *et al.* Promoting quality: the health-care organization from a management perspective. *International Journal for Quality in Health Care.* 2007; **19**: 341–8.

102 Ferlie EB, Shortell SM. Improving the quality of health care in the United Kingdom and the United States: a framework for change. *The Milbank Quarterly.* 2000; **79**: 281.

103 Rogers E. *Diffusion of Innovations.* 5th ed. New York: The Free Press; 2003.

104 Dowling B, Powell M, Glendinning C. *Health and Social Care in the Community.* 2004; **12**: 309–17.

105 Hernandez SR. Horizontal and vertical integration: lessons learned from the United States. *HealthcarePapers.* 2000; **1**: 59–65.

106 Shortell, SM, Gillies R, Devers K. Reinventing the American hospital. *The Milbank Quarterly.* 1995; **73**: 131–60.

107 Himmelman A. Coalitions and the transformation of power relations: collaborative betterment and collaborative empowerment. *American Journal of Community Psychology.* 2001; **29**: 277–84.

108 Joyce AS, Wild TC, Adair CE, *et al.* Continuity of care in mental health services: toward clarifying the construct. *Canadian Journal of Psychiatry.* 2004; **49**: 539–50.

109 Midgely G. Systems thinking in evaluation. In: Williams B, Iman I, editors. *Systems Concepts in Evaluation: an expert anthology.* Battle Creek, MI: Kellogg Foundation; 2007. pp. 11–34.

110 Foster-Fishman P, Nowell B, Yang H. Putting the system back into systems change: a framework for understanding and changing organizational and community systems. *American Journal of Psychology.* 2007; **39**: 197–215.

111 Olney CA. Using evaluation to adapt health information outreach to the complex environments of community-based organizations. *Journal of the Medical Library Association.* 2005; **93**(Suppl. 4): S57–67.

112 Wheatley M, Frieze D. *Lifecycle of Emergence: using emergence to take social innovations to scale.* The Berkana Institute; 2006. Available at: www.berkana.org/articles/lifecycle.htm (accessed 7 July 2010).

113 Singer HH, Kegler MC. Assessing interorganizational networks as a dimension of community capacity: illustrations from a community intervention to prevent lead poisoning. *Health Education & Behavior.* 2004; **31**: 808–21.

114 Brass DJ, Galaskiewicz J, Greve HR, *et al.* Taking stock of networks and organizations: a multilevel perspective. *Academy of Management Journal.* 2004; **47**: 795–817.

115 Tausig M. Detecting 'cracks' in mental health service systems: application of network analytic techniques. *American Journal of Community Psychology.* 1987; **15**: 337–51.

116 Morrissey JP, Calloway MO, Thakur N, *et al.* Integration of service systems for homeless persons with serious mental illness through the ACCESS program. *Psychiatric Services.* 2003; **53**: 949–57.

117 Provan KG, Milward HB. A preliminary theory of interorganizational network effectiveness: a comparative study of four community mental health systems. *Administrative Science Quarterly.* 1995; **40**: 1–33.

118 Walker R. *Collaboration and Alliances: a review for VicHealth.* Victoria, BC: VicHealth; 2000.

119 Williams B, Imanv I, editors. *Systems Concepts in Evaluation: an expert anthology.* Battle Creek, MI: Kellogg Foundation; 2007.

120 Barlow DH. Psychological treatments. *American Journal of Psychology.* 2004; **59**: 869–78.

121 Castonguay LG, Beutler LE. Principles of therapeutic change: a task force on participants, relationships, and techniques factors. *Journal of Clinical Psychology.* 2006; **62**: 631–8.

122 Asay, TP, Lambert, MJ. The empirical case for the common factors in therapy: quantitative findings. In: Hubble MA, Duncan BL, editors. *The Heart and Soul of Change: what works in therapy.* Washington, DC: American Psychological Association; 1999. pp. 23–55.

123 Beutler LE, Malik M, Alimohamed S, *et al.* Therapist variables. In: Lambert MH, editor. *Handbook of Psychotherapy and Behaviour Change.* 5th ed. New York: Wiley; 2003. pp. 227–306.

124 Ilgen MA, McKellar J, Moos R, *et al.* Therapeutic alliance and the relationship between motivation and treatment outcomes in patients with alcohol use disorder. *Journal of Substance Abuse Treatment.* 2006; **31**: 157–62.

125 Morgenstern J, McKay JR. Rethinking the paradigms that inform behavioral treatment research for substance use disorders. *Addiction.* 2007; **102**: 1377–89.

126 Baldwin SA, Wampold BE, Imel ZE. Untangling the alliance-outcome correlation: exploring the relative importance of therapist and patient variability in the alliance. *Journal of Consulting and Clinical Psychology.* 2007; **75**: 842–52.

127 Anderson T, Ogles BM, Patterson CL, *et al.* Therapist effects: facilitative interpersonal skills as a predictor of therapist success. *Journal of Clinical Psychology.* 2009; **65**: 755–68.

128 Bertrand K, Nadeau L. Toxicomanie et inadaptation sociale grave: perspectives subjectives de femmes en traitement quant à l'initiation et la progression de leur consommation. *Drogues, Santé et Société.* 2006; **5**: 9–44.

TO LEARN MORE

- For links to resources and training related to mental health–substance use disorders: www.camh.net/
- For links to resources and access to expertise and consultation related to integration of mental health and substance use services: www.zialogic.org/
- For links to resources on substance use services and systems in Canada, including mental health and substance use: www.ccsa.ca and www.ccsa.ca/ceca/

CHAPTER 13

Mental health–substance use in emergency settings

Salena Williams

INTRODUCTION

Assessment, treatment and care of the individual experiencing mental health–substance use problems, presenting to the emergency department (ED) of a general hospital, is part of the liaison psychiatry team's everyday clinical practice. A large percentage of psychiatric presentations to the ED involve substance use. Many people who we see use substances in their everyday lives: to find some enjoyment, to blot out the upset in their lives, to act as a solution for problems, or as part of overdose either to expedite the process of the poisons, or to enable the individual to build up the courage needed to attempt suicide. The ED of an inner-city general hospital in some ways mirrors the lifestyle of the person experiencing mental health–substance use problems. It is home to intermittent chaos and efficiency, a mix of complex needs, and holds within it people in crisis – both physical and psychological.

REFLECTIVE PRACTICE EXERCISE 13.1 – SEE P. 188 FOR ANSWERS

> **Time: 10 minutes**
> Alcohol, and to a lesser extent drugs, are everywhere, readily available. They complicate everything that presents to us in the ED.
> - Think about the ways in which a low-stimulus environment can alter the relationship created with the individual, and how a low-stimulus environment could be created in ED.
> - What other professional communication techniques could help the individual's experience?

KEY POINT 13.1 RISK ASSESSMENT AT TRIAGE

The NICE guidelines for self-harm recommend that all individuals with mental health needs should have access to a mental health assessment.[1] Developing a triage tool such as the Australasian triage system,[2] or the Risk Assessment Matrix,[3] allows ED professionals to assess mental state on admission and indicate on referral to the psychiatric liaison team the level of risk and therefore the urgency of referral response.

LIAISON PSYCHIATRY IN THE EMERGENCY DEPARTMENT

Liaison psychiatry professionals are specialist mental health workers in the ED and hold a unique role in the assessment and treatment of the individual experiencing mental health–substance use problems. On receipt of referral, information from diverse sources (from carers, across the mental health trust, social services, primary care) is collated in a timely way.[4] Assessments can be swift yet all encompassing, including accurate assessment of risk. The liaison psychiatry team is multidisciplinary so that a holistic view of care is taken, and the diversity of presentation is effectively assessed and treated.

Harm reduction is part of the public health agenda.[5] The individual experiencing substance use, and mental and physical ill health presenting at ED gives a unique opportunity for education and awareness raising, both in terms of control of infection, and psychological support.

Awareness of problems, such as foetal alcohol syndrome, infected groin injection or needle sharing can allow the individual to make informed choices about their substance use. A good evidence-based practice model is the combination of psychiatric liaison professionals and substance use specialist professionals. Hospital-based bacteraemia is problematic, and drug users have been identified as a group more at risk, but also more likely to bring blood-borne infection into the hospital environment. Drug and alcohol specialist nurses are key to this process, shaping the environment and providing a seamless service from hospital to community. A good liaison psychiatry service would have drug and alcohol specialist nurses attached to it, working jointly as necessary. Protocols for titration of detoxification regimes and appropriate prescribing regimes for those with drug addiction should be available in ED. Alcohol specialist nurses are also key to streamlining and specialising care in the ED. Joint assessments and team working closely with specialist nurses help to enable the individual to have access to psychological support, and appropriate community follow-up according to the emphasis of their diagnosis, i.e. what the person sees as their main problem.

Case study 13.1

A 54-year-old man:

* unemployed, homeless
* previous diagnosis of bipolar illness, had been treated by community mental health team but lost contact
* past history of severe physical and sexual abuse
* guilt about his own paedophilic urges
* past history of severe self-mutilation

- drinks alcohol: one and a half bottles of whisky per day
- wants to die.

This gentleman was admitted after falling from a cliff in a nearby wooded area. It transpired that he had purposefully jumped from the cliff in an attempt to end his life, and had spent some time before the suicide attempt sending letters to his brother and ex-wife to apologise and say goodbye. He exhibited symptoms of alcohol intoxication and was vulnerable to exploitation by others. A homelessness health nurse was an invaluable source of support for him, and information for the psychiatric liaison team. After assessment of his mental state, he was admitted to hospital for treatment of his fractured tibia, and assessed under the UK Mental Health Act,[6] and detained under Section 2. He was later transferred to a psychiatric ward.

KEY POINT 13.2 USING THE MENTAL HEALTH ACT IN THE EMERGENCY DEPARTMENT

Most sections of the Mental Health Act[6] do not apply to the emergency department. A person in ED is not admitted to hospital, therefore only the Section 136 (in which police will bring the individual into ED for medical treatment while exercising their holding power) or Section 4 for emergency medical treatment will be seen – and this is rarely used. The Mental Health Act[6] cannot be used in the context of a primary drug or alcohol problem. Once admitted to a hospital ward, clinicians could consider using Section 5(2) of the Act to detain the individual while awaiting mental health assessment.

PSYCHOSOCIAL ASSESSMENT IN THE EMERGENCY DEPARTMENT

One of the primary ways in which we have contact with the individual experiencing mental health–substance use problems is as suicide attempters or self-harm person attending the ED. Appleby's seminal confidential enquiry[7] revealed that individuals experiencing mental health–substance use problems are not only more likely to harm others but to self-harm. Self-harm while acutely intoxicated is of no less risk than those who are not using substances. Anecdotally, up to 80% of overdoses have used alcohol before taking the overdose: be that as a precursor to the suicidal thoughts – '*there was nothing wrong with me during the day, then later in the night I began to think life wasn't worth living*' (person's self-report), as a 'courage' style form of relaxing the self to take the action, or as a deliberate choice of expedient of the overdose.

A standardised assessment compliant with UK NICE guidelines for self-harm[1] is essential in the assessment process. Assessment will include:

➤ a mental state examination

> a full history – including family, personal, drug and alcohol, forensic
> the circumstances of the event that preceded hospital admission.

Assessment would also include contact with statutory/voluntary services in the past, medical conditions and a risk screen itemising epidemiological risk factors (*see* Book 5, Chapters 7, 8, 9).

The ED assessment takes place in isolation of social and personal circumstances. This can be a useful exchange, providing a new perspective on problems that may have been long-standing. However, in the absence of previous information the interview must be accurate and all encompassing, especially about consumption of drugs or alcohol. Acute confusion mistaken for intoxication can be potentially fatal. While the individual is intoxicated they may not be able to give a full history, and vital parts of the assessment may be missed due to lack of available information from other sources. For example, if homeless, the individual may have accessed several general practitioners. Many symptoms of psychiatric illness may be misunderstood, or misdiagnosed as the effects of substance use. Serious and potentially life-threatening consequences of alcohol use, such as delirium tremens and Wernicke's syndrome, can be missed. Benzodiazepine withdrawal can mimic some symptoms of anxiety or psychotic illness. Collateral information whenever possible – from partner, friends, carer, key worker – can also be vital at the assessment stage.

KEY POINT 13.3 RECOGNISING ALCOHOL WITHDRAWAL

The main symptoms to look for are as follows:
- tremor
- sweating
- nausea/'dry heaves'
- anxiety
- irritability
- restlessness
- unexplained grand-mal seizure.

More severe signs and symptoms which indicate delirium tremens include:
- confusion
- auditory and visual hallucinations
- extreme fear/agitation
- disorientation.

In an alcohol-dependent individual where there is usually high tolerance to alcohol, withdrawal symptoms may be present well before the blood alcohol is negative.

Abnormal liver function results are useful in highlighting alcohol misuse/dependence. If concerned, ensure the hospital's alcohol protocol is followed. Ensure the use of high levels of prophylactic parenteral vitamin B if there is a suspicion of alcohol use.

Once the detoxification process is complete, there should be a further mental state assessment to exclude the presence of more serious mental illness, e.g. the psychotic symptoms may still be present and, thus, could be part of a hitherto untreated psychotic illness.

Parenting may be affected by substance use or mental health problems. There may be risk issues around the use of medication or weapons for self-harm that may affect the psychological well-being or physical safety of the child/children. Safeguarding children who may be at risk is part of person-centred care and treatment. Children can be referred to social services as a 'child of concern'. It is important that this is explained to the individual, and any anxieties about possibly 'losing' their children to social services be talked through (*see* Chapter 7).

Case study 13.2

A 37-year-old woman:

- threatened partner with a knife in the context of heavy alcohol use
- threatened to kill herself with the same knife
- the partner smashed her head against the pavement outside their home
- police were called to the incident; they then called an ambulance
- she was complaining of headache, had suffered severe nose bleeds for the past three months
- reported periods of 'going blind'.

This woman was assessed by the staff grade medical doctor in ED, who reported the symptoms as 'just alcohol-related'. The psychiatric liaison nurse was asked to assess her due to the suicidal ideation voiced at the scene of the assault. In the course of the psychiatric assessment, the individual reported no peripheral vision. The psychiatric nurse reported this, and requested further neurological investigations. On the magnetic resonance imaging (MRI) scan she was found to have central frontal injury to her brain. Full investigations were then completed, and appropriate physical treatment given (*see* Chapter 17).

In England, emergency departments have a current – possibly soon to change – political and cost-led agenda of four hours to see, treat and discharge the individual, which leads to a tightly structured organisational design. Speed of response to each individual is crucial to the running of the ED. Because of the rapidity of the referral and interaction, there is scant opportunity for flexibility in the care pathway, or innovative approaches to care. There is a medical emphasis to triage and physical assessments can be in busy minor or major injury areas. The individual is surrounded by medical equipment offering access to potential weapons of self-harm, or others in the area, for example needles, oxygen flex, or hand cleansers that can be drunk for the alcohol content. The emergency nature of the admission means that the person usually brings very little information with them. The individual experiencing mental health–substance use problems may have repeated attendances, sometimes spending twice as many days in hospital than those with mental health problems but no substance use.[8] Many of these individuals will be actively under the influence of drugs/alcohol and may present as a management risk, or as an 'unpopular patient'.[9] These individuals are often the butt of double stigma (*see* Book 1, Chapters 4, 5, 7): ignorance and prejudice and expected set of behaviours based on myths around both mental ill health and substance use. Stigma is still prevalent in the general public and among professionals about both mental health and substance use, ranging from benevolence to fear, exclusion and negative stereotyping.[10]

Assessment may be difficult due to the level of intoxication, both acutely and chronically, affecting the ability to work alongside the individual psychologically or via medication use. The person may exacerbate the dynamic by expressing violent and aggressive behaviour or language. There may be intervention by hospital security, ejection from the hospital before treatment is completed, or the person may take his/her own discharge before being seen.

Individuals using substances may present as challenging to the mental health professional as they are perceived to have no motivation to stop and elicit the thought that 'we cannot do anything', that 'we are powerlessness to help'. However, individuals who present to ED experiencing mental health–substance use problems give hospital professionals an opportunity for medical assessment and intervention, as well as a chance to gain a psychological assessment and possibly effect behaviour change.

SELF-ASSESSMENT EXERCISE 13.1

Time: 15 minutes

Mental health–substance use problems present the individual in ED with a 'double stigma': that of mental ill health ('he's just crazy') and using a 'vice substance' deserving of punishment. It is worth considering our own drug, alcohol and lifestyle habits:

- Should being overweight mean that the individual is less deserving of treatment or care?
- Should smoking or not smoking be a decision maker with regards having heart bypass operations?
- What factors would indicate a label 'problem patient' to you?
- What are the ethical implications?
- Would this be acceptable to you, or your relative?

EDUCATION AND CONSULTATION ROLE OF LIAISON PSYCHIATRY

Combating stigma can be achieved within the ED itself by providing role modelling to nursing and medical staff. It may involve challenging adverse reactions on the spot. There is an important role to be played by liaison psychiatry in the general hospital in teaching both informally and formally, to raise awareness and recognition of illness and distress suffered by the individual experiencing mental health problems who also uses substances. Inclusion of the individual who has experienced mental health–substance use problems in the training of professionals can have dramatic impact on care. These individuals can be instrumental in the review of operations, and can be involved in the hospital's Mental Health Operational Group, and ultimately help to shape service provision.

Case study 13.3

Inappropriate opiate use of asylum-seeking woman with sickle cell anemia.
   A 28-year-old woman:
- originally from Jamaica
- asylum seeker
- witness to death of brothers
- given one year for medical health issues to be addressed
- no family in UK
- living with violent partner
- sickle cell illness
- intermittent pain to limbs
- multiple admissions to hospital
- tearful, poor sleep
- frequently leaving the ward especially at night
- frequent overt requests for opiates and benzodiazepines.

A joint mental health assessment revealed details of sexual abuse in childhood and traumatic incidents in Jamaica. Women's refuge contacted and new anonymous housing was provided. Sickle cell association locally was contacted to help with reducing social isolation. She was referred to psychology outpatients for further assessment and psychological input for stress/pain relationship and trauma experiences. Antidepressant medication was prescribed via the general practitioner.

Depression and anxiety are common in people with physical illness. They may use drugs or alcohol to cope with feelings of low mood, worthlessness, panic attacks or poor sleep. Depression or anxiety are sometimes missed in people with physical health problems as it is assumed that to be down or anxious because you are ill is normal, not pathological. This is not the case. Many people with physical illness are resilient, even happy, and coping or adapting well to their illness. Depression or anxiety may be a consequence of the illness, or physical illness and anxiety/depression may be aetiologically distinct. Substance use may predate the onset of the physical illness, and may be the causative factor of the depression. Substance use may also be a risk factor in exacerbation of the physical illness, such as pancreatitis. Depression and anxiety may affect the rehabilitation from an illness, or may exacerbate drug use.[11]

Accurate assessment of the depression or anxiety is crucial. This can be done using an evidence-based tool such as Beck's depression inventory.[12] Ideally, there needs to be a period of abstinence to get clear diagnosis of depression. It may be that in the case of anxiety, the drug or alcohol use needs to be treated in the first instance, before the anxiety can be successfully treated.[13] Antidepressant medication can be helpful in reducing symptoms of depression and alcohol consumption. However, diagnosis of depression becomes much more complex while someone is using alcohol due to depressive effects of the alcohol itself.

PSYCHOLOGICAL TREATMENT IN THE EMERGENCY DEPARTMENT

Psychological approaches in the ED can be effective. Empathic listening to a person's beliefs about their illness and prognosis can be helpful, as well as brief interventions (*see* Book 4, Chapter 8; Book 5, Chapter 10), such as problem-solving.

KEY POINT 13.4 PROBLEM-SOLVING

Problem-solving[14] is not a complex form of psychological intervention and can easily be cascaded to colleagues.

- Ask the individual to define and list their current problems.
- Choose a problem for action.
- List alternative courses of action (including outlandish ideas such as taking a rocket to the moon!). This can introduce humour but also widen horizons and encourage more imaginative possible solutions.
- Evaluate courses of action and choose the best.
- Engage the individual in trying out the action.
- Evaluate the results.
- Repeat this process on all problems listed.

Some evidence suggests that short psychological interventions can be effective in the hospital setting in reducing and stopping alcohol use.[15,16] Professionals working in liaison psychiatry are experts at rapid engagement with newly referred individuals.

In some respects, a large part of the assessment process is motivational interviewing (*see* Book 4, Chapter 7). Mental health assessment would routinely include how much alcohol/drugs the individual has consumed in the 48 hours previous to hospital admission as part of the suicide risk assessment. Reviewing the circumstances surrounding hospital admission may allow the individual to begin assessment of their substance use and to recognise early warning signs of relapse (*see* Book 6, Chapters 15, 16).

Benefits of treatment with antidepressants are many, including improved quality of life, and improved compliance with medical treatment. However, although it is important that the person receives treatment for depression quickly, it must be borne in mind that some medications carry an early risk of suicidal ideation, especially with younger people. It is important that medications are not prescribed from ED, and that individuals are encouraged to discuss the use of antidepressants with their general practitioner on discharge from hospital so that stepped care[18] and longer-term monitoring is achieved. The general practitioner may be a key source for providing assessment of, and access to, psychological treatments for things which may have triggered substance use problem, such as traumatic events or bereavement (*see* Chapters 10 and 11), for example a soldier who has become depressed and a heavy alcohol drinker due to the symptoms of post-traumatic stress disorder (*see* Book 6, Chapter 9). Education and reassurance about common reactions to bereavement, loss or threats to self, associated with physical illness can be useful.

SELF-HELP

Self-help (*see* Book 4, Chapters 14 and 15) can play an important part in empowering people to look at and find their own solutions. In Bristol, England, a *Services to Help You* leaflet is distributed to all individuals. It is supported by the hospital, and designed to look similar to other booklets such as *Head Injury Services to Help You* to reduce stigma. The leaflet for people using substances includes:
➤ health awareness
➤ information about risks
➤ nutritional information
➤ reducing infection.

Substance use is commonly associated with increased hospital admission, relapse in physical illness, and poor health generally.

NON-STATUTORY AGENCIES

Non-statutory agencies can be more accessible, as they are self-referral and offer voluntary admission. Examples of these are the Addiction Recovery Agency, Alcoholics Anonymous and Narcotics Anonymous, as well as voluntary sector substance use agencies. Many voluntary sector services offer one-to-one support, out of hours support, accommodation or rehabilitation, and long-term help that statutory services are no longer able to offer. Alcoholics Anonymous may offer an onsite hospital group.

In Bristol, individuals of suicide or mental health low risk who are discharged by an ED professional following triage assessment using the Risk Assessment Matrix[3] are encouraged to attend the outpatient self-harm clinic and given an appointment letter, in a similar manner to those returning to the trauma clinic or other outpatients clinics. In this way, the aim is to integrate mental health and substance use services with other hospital users.

BARRIERS TO CARE

There are barriers when referring to appropriate agencies on discharge. Discharge from ED can be delayed by lack of ownership of those who are experiencing mental health–substance use problems. Lack of coordination and integration of services and a confusing array of service provision may mean that some people are at risk of 'falling through the net'. Some are at that point of wanting to change – to stop using alcohol or drugs – but are unable to find or gain access to a rapid response service to go with that, and return to the corner shop or drug dealer, with loss of momentum and loss of impetus to change. Sectorisation of services has led to boundaried care. It is crucial in the assessment process to establish the primary problem at the time of attendance in hospital so that appropriate follow-up is ensured. There is a danger that individuals can become a 'bouncing ball' between mental health and substance use services. Whenever the person is under existing services, joint assessments with Community Psychiatric Nurses, outreach workers and/or homelessness workers can increase the streamlining and coordination of care.

CONCLUSION

Presentations of mental ill health and substance use are common in the emergency department setting. Commonly, individuals will present in crisis, either with self-harm or as a result of physical illness related to substance use. It is important that the individual receives equitable care and is listened to. Skilful and meaningful psychosocial assessment and treatment at this 'magical moment', a window of opportunity due to hospitalisation, can change lives and even save lives.

ANSWER TO REFLECTIVE PRACTICE EXERCISE 13.1

- Consistency of the professionals.
- Clear, short explanations and reassurance.
- Ensuring adequate hydration.
- Observe for signs/symptoms of hostility or responding to hallucinations/ delusions.

REFERENCES

1 National Institute of Clinical Excellence. *Self-harm: the short-term physical and psychological management and secondary prevention of self-harm in primary and secondary care.* NICE guidance 16. London: NIHCE; 2004. Available at: www.nice.org.uk/nicemedia/pdf/ CG016NICEguideline.pdf (accessed 8 July 2010).

2 Australasian College of Emergency Medicine. *Guidelines for the Implementation of the Australasian Triage Scale in Emergency Departments.* Carlton, VIC: Australasian College of Emergency Medicine; 2000.

3 Hart C, Colley R, Harrison A. Using a risk assessment matrix with mental health patients in emergency departments. *Emergency Nurse.* 2005; **12**: 21–8.

4 O'Keefe N, Ramaiah E, Nomani M, *et al.* Benchmarking a liaison psychiatry service: a prospective 6 month study of quality indicators. *Psychiatric Bulletin.* 2007: **31**: 345–7.

5 Bristol Partnership. *Bristol Harm Reduction Strategy.* Bristol: Bristol Partnership; 2008. Available at: www.bristol.gov.uk/ccm/content/Community-Living/Crime-Prevention/safer-bristol-partnership/alcohol-harm-reduction-strategy (accessed 8 July 2010).

6 Department of Health. *Mental Health Act 2007.* Available at: www.opsi.gov.uk/acts/ acts2007/pdf/ukpga_20070012_en.pdf (accessed 8 July 2010).

7 Appleby L. Safer services: conclusions from the report of the National Confidential Enquiry. *Advances in Psychiatric Treatment.* 2000; **1**: 5–15.

8 Menezes P, Johnson S, Thornicroft G, *et al.* Drug and alcohol problems among individuals with severe mental illness in south London. *British Journal of Psychiatry.* 1996; **168**: 612–19.

9 Johnson M, Webb C. Rediscovering the unpopular patient: the concept of social judgement. *Journal of Advanced Nursing.* 2006; **21**: 466–75.

10 Byrne P. Psychiatric stigma. *British Journal of Psychiatry.* 2001; **178**: 281–4.

11 Rounsaville B. Treatment of cocaine dependence and depression. *Biological Psychiatry*. 2004; **56**: 803–9.

12 Beck A, Steer R, Ball R, *et al*. Comparison of Beck depression inventories -IA and -II in psychiatric outpatients. *Journal of Personality Assessment*. 1996; **67**: 588–97.

13 Lingford-Hughes A, Potokar J, Nutt D. Treating anxiety complicated by substance misuse. *Advances in Psychiatric Treatment*. 2002; **8**: 107–16.

14 Wright B, Williams C, Garland A. Using the five areas cognitive-behavioural model with psychiatric patients. *Advances in Psychiatric Treatment*. 2002; **8**: 307–15.

15 Love A, Greenberg M, Brice M, *et al*. Emergency department screening and intervention for patients with alcohol-related disorders: a pilot study. *Journal of American Osteopathic Association*. 2008; **108**: 12–20.

16 Crawford M, Patton R, Touquet R. Screening and referral for brief intervention of alcohol-misusing patients in an emergency department: a pragmatic randomized controlled trial. *Lancet*. 2004; **364**: 1334–9.

17 Rollnick S, Miller W, Butler C. *Motivational Interviewing in Healthcare: helping patients change behaviour*. London: Guildford Press; 2007.

18 Bower P, Gilbody S. Stepped care in psychological therapies: access effectiveness and efficiency. *British Journal of Psychiatry*. 2005; **186**: 11–17.

TO LEARN MORE

- British Pain Society. *Pain and Substance Misuse: improving the patient experience*. London: The British Pain Society; 2007.
- Grenberger D, Padesky C. *Mind over Mood*. London: Guildford Press; 1995.
- Health Protection Agency. *Shooting Up: infections among drug users in the United Kingdom 2007*. London: Health Protection Agency; 2008.
- MacHale S. Managing depression in physical illness. *Advances in Psychiatric Treatment*. 2002; **8**: 287–306.
- Department of Health and the devolved administrations. *Drug Misuse and Dependence: UK guidelines on clinical management* [The Orange Guidelines]. London: Department of Health (England), the Scottish Government, Welsh Assembly Government and Northern Ireland Executive; 2007. Available at: www.nta.nhs.uk/publications/documents/clinical_guidelines_2007.pdf
- Regel S, Roberts D. *Liaison Psychiatry: a handbook for nurses and health professionals*. London: Elsevier Health Services; 2002.
- Royal College of Physicians Royal College of Psychiatrists. *The Psychological Care of Medical Patients: a practical guide*. London: Royal College Physicians, Royal College of Psychiatrists; 2003.
- Stern TA, Fricchione GL, Cassem NH, *et al*., editors. *Massachusetts General Hospital Handbook of General Hospital Psychiatry*. 5th ed. Philadelphia, PA: Mosby; 2004.
- BBC Headroom: www.bbc.co.uk/headroom/newsandevents/recomreads.shtml
- Understanding the psychological effects of street drugs. Mind Booklet. Available at: www.mind.org.uk/shop/booklets/diagnoses_treatment/509_understanding_the_psychological_effects_of_street_drugs

CHAPTER 14

Crime, prison, mental health–substance use

Lisa Blecha, Michael Lukasiewicz and Michel Reynaud

CHAPTER LEARNING OBJECTIVES

To understand:

➤ current epidemiology of mental illness–substance use disorders in prison
➤ people to watch for; the most 'needy'
➤ effective and validated screening tools in the prison setting
➤ current treatment initiatives in and after prisons
➤ specific prisoners and their needs (women, juvenile offenders) and to think about future programmes of treatment.

WHAT IS KNOWN ABOUT THE EPIDEMIOLOGY OF MENTAL HEALTH–SUBSTANCE USE DISORDERS IN PRISON?

Mental illness among people in prison is highly prevalent. The UK Office for National Statistics has shown that the risk of affective and anxiety disorders is approximately three times that in the British general population, of personality disorder 13 times and of schizophrenia 16 times.[1]

A meta-analysis among 23 000 European prisoners has shown prevalences of 4% for psychotic disorders, 10% affective disorders and 65% personality disorders (47% antisocial disorder), in men. In total, one prisoner in seven has either a psychotic or a major depressive disorder and one prisoner in two has a personality disorder.[1]

To translate this into 'real' figures, conservative estimates in the United States show a total of approximately 450 000 prisoners with any mental condition and 322 000 prisoners with severe mental illness in US jails, state and federal prisons.[2]

Several studies have shown that mental health–substance use is a significant problem in prison. According to US Department of Justice figures, approximately 75% of prisoners who had mental illness also met criteria for substance use disorder. Inversely, 63% of those who had a substance use disorder also met criteria for mental illness.[3]

People in prison experiencing mental disorders would also seem to have a history of chronic instability and difficulties adapting to life in society.[4] A significantly greater proportion of prisoners with mental illness have a history of homelessness prior to their arrest and have difficulties adapting to the prison environment with violations of facility rules (58% versus 43%) and injuries in altercations with others (20% versus 10%).[5,6] Box 14.1 shows a typical profile of a prisoner experiencing mental illness.

BOX 14.1 Typical profile of a prisoner experiencing mental illness

- Young (under 30)
- Three or more prior incarcerations
- Recent homelessness
- Family history of substance use disorder
- 'Troublemaker' or 'scapegoat' with difficulties adapting to the prison environment
- Isolation inside and outside prison (few prison visits, loner), frequent disciplinary sanctions
- Low level of education, few job skills.

The person in prison with the greatest mental healthcare needs is probably the one who is the hardest to reach due to poorly adapted and/or aggressive behaviour in and out of the prison environment, and who is frequently isolated due to their behaviour.

DO MENTALLY ILL AND NON-MENTALLY ILL PEOPLE PERCEIVE PRISON DIFFERENTLY?

Very little is known about the subjective experience of people in prison, and even less is known about the specific factors related to perception differences. Imprisonment was conceived as a humane alternative to corporal punishment. Punishment to the 'soul' or mind was conceived to atone for wrongs done instead of inflicting physical pain. To date, few studies have examined the interpretation that people in prison attribute to the prison experience and if this interpretation could be different in certain sub-groups, such as people experiencing mental disorders.

A recent study in a French population of prisoners condemned to long-term sentences has shown that mentally ill prisoners use more hostile terms to describe prison conditions.[7] Mentally ill people describe imprisonment in terms of persecution and often attribute their suffering to external circumstances. These feelings may increase following disciplinary actions, such as isolation and confinement which are more frequent in the mentally ill. These actions may also increase feelings of helplessness and victimisation in this population. Feelings of persecution may lead to violent reactions. Thus, a person experiencing mental health disorders may be trapped in an unending circle of increasing violence followed by increasingly harsh reprimands.

For these reasons, it is important to screen prisoners for mental health–substance use disorders. Individuals can be oriented towards appropriate treatment programmes and prison living conditions.

KEY POINT 14.1

Acting out, excessive reactions to minor incidents could be a sign that the person feels persecuted. Further psychiatric evaluation may be warranted.

EVALUATING AND SCREENING FOR MENTAL HEALTH–SUBSTANCE USE DISORDER

One of the key criteria defined in the Trenčín[8] statement on prisons and mental health is the necessity for each individual to be fully assessed for their mental and physical health needs on entering the prison environment. Prisons are often under-staffed with numerous prisoners to be seen. Any systematic screening must respond to a certain number of criteria:

➤ acceptable to prison officers and the individual
➤ practical – deliver a maximum amount of information within a minimum amount of time
➤ valid and reliable.

Screening instruments should be usable by professionals who do not necessarily have any formal psychiatric training, but who must decide whether to refer the individual for further psychiatric evaluation or for immediate treatment (*see* Box 14.2).

BOX 14.2 Initial screening instruments validated for mental health–substance use disorders

Mental illness screening
- Referral Decision Scale (RDS): some validity issues (excessive false positives)[9,10]
- Brief Jail Mental Health Screen (BJMHS): eight items, administration: 2–5 minutes[9]
- Screening Instrument for Psychosis.[11]

Substance use screening
- Simple Screening Instrument-Substance Abuse (SSI-SA)[12]
- Texas Christian University Drug Screen (TCUDS)[13]
- Alcohol Dependence Scale (ADS).[14]

Each instrument can be used by prison personnel with minimal training. The questions are simple and adapted to anyone with a minimal level of education. In the case of the mental illness screens, their purpose is to exclude the most serious psychiatric symptoms in order to refer people as quickly as possible to appropriate treatment programmes. Given the limited number of psychiatrists and psychiatric nurses in the prison setting, only those individuals who have the most urgent needs should be referred.

The substance use screens are primarily used to determine if a person would need to be referred for appropriate substance use counselling. Other more elaborate screens exist, but they require trained personnel to administer and interpret the results.

REFERRAL FOR ACUTE WITHDRAWAL SYMPTOMS

All prison personnel should be trained to recognise acute withdrawal symptoms and to refer the individuals for medical care when necessary. Sedative, alcohol and opiate withdrawal is associated with adrenergic symptoms or signs of stress.

KEY POINT 14.2

Alcohol, sedative and opiate withdrawal signs. Watch out for the person who 'SwEARS'.

- **Sw**eating, shaking
- **E**yes: wide open, anxious, watchful, pupils dilated
- **A**nxiety: heart racing
- **R**ush, redness
- **S**eeing things.

Individuals showing signs of acute withdrawal should be immediately referred for medical treatment. Serious acute alcohol and sedative withdrawal can rapidly evolve towards epileptic seizures that could prove fatal. Medical management using benzodiazepines and sufficient hydration can prevent seizures and hallucinations, or at least limit their consequences. If signs of withdrawal are observed, the individual should be moved to a calm area and monitored carefully until the medical team arrives to evaluate and treat him.

On the other end of the spectrum, stimulants, such as cocaine and amphetamines, may also cause a certain number of withdrawal signs.

KEY POINT 14.3

Signs of stimulant withdrawal (cocaine, amphetamines). Watch out for the 'LIFELESS' person.

- **L**istlessness
- **I**ncreased appetite
- **F**atigue
- **E**xtenuation
- **Le**thargy
- **S**uicidal thoughts and **S**uicidal plans
- **D**ifficulties concentrating
- **D**epression which may be serious (melancholic).

Only melancholy with suicidal intent represents a life-threatening situation that must be recognised and treated. The other situations are dangerous because of decreased awareness and capacity to judge. Elaborate preventive action is needed as the situation requires. This could leave these individuals victims to violence and aggression from other prisoners. People who seem to be sad and listless should be questioned concerning suicidal thoughts and plans. Such individuals should be rapidly referred for a more complete psychiatric evaluation.

SPECIFIC MANAGEMENT OF SUBSTANCE USE-DEPENDENT INDIVIDUALS

Opiate substitution treatment

Opiate substitution treatment varies among countries. One of the most common treatments is methadone. Methadone acts as a slow-acting opiate receptor agonist that eliminates the symptoms of opiate withdrawal, but does not cause signs of intoxication and sedation. It can be used in combination with numerous other treatments such as neuroleptics. It can also be used with addictolytic medications such as acamprosate.

KEY POINT 14.4

Buprenorphine must not be used with opiate antagonists, such as naltrexone, that precipitate opiate withdrawal symptoms.

Care should also be taken when methadone is used with benzodiazepines since sedative effects from both drugs could be increased. Doses should be started at 30–40 mg once daily and gradually increased by 10 mg every two days until withdrawal signs disappear. Doses can be increased up to 180 mg per day.

In certain countries, buprenorphine substitution treatment is also available. Buprenorphine is a partial opiate receptor agonist. In France, buprenorphine has been available since 1996. It can be prescribed by the general practitioner on a secure prescription pad. Because of its agonist/antagonist properties, people must be warned against using other opiates when taking buprenorphine. Simultaneous use can cause acute opiate withdrawal symptoms. The particular pharmacological profile for buprenorphine also prevents overdose. Once the receptors are blocked, excess buprenorphine is eliminated. Treatment can be instigated at a dose of 4–6 mg per day and increased by 2 mg every two days until there are no signs of withdrawal. The maximum recommended dose for buprenorphine is 16 mg per day.

Acute setting

Heroin withdrawal is particularly difficult, especially during a short-term imprisonment. The individual may be particularly anxious, due to her/his transitory and uncertain situation. Anxiety in addition to substance cravings can make withdrawal difficult. Certain individuals dependent on substances may become irritable, causing them to act out at the slightest incident. In addition to adrenal 'SwEARS' signs, heroin withdrawal has the specificity of causing lower back and joint pains, tearing and nasal drip. People may experience diarrhoea and abdominal cramps.

These symptoms are reduced by the administration of an opiate substitute, such as buprenorphine or methadone.

These individuals should be rapidly seen by a physician and short-term opiate substitution treatment proposed. They should be moved to a calm, isolated area and carefully monitored until the physician arrives. It is important to carefully note any prior opiate substitution prescriptions and other medications and substances currently used. These can also cause withdrawal signs and can aggravate the overall situation.

Long-term setting

Opiate substitution policies in prisons vary worldwide. Some countries, such as the United States, are just beginning to experiment with methadone treatment a few days prior to release. In France, methadone or buprenorphine substitution is available. Research has shown that prison-based treatment for substance use problems has a favourable impact on the individual's transition to life outside of prison. Methadone treatment has also been associated with less drug use outside of prison as shown by fewer opiate-positive urine screens.[15,16] In addition, opiate substitution treatment has a favourable impact with lesser human immunodeficiency virus (HIV) and hepatitis C virus (HCV) transmission due to syringe and material sharing.[17,18]

DRUG TREATMENT IN PRISON: DOES IT WORK?

As shown in a 1998 report for the Office of National Drug Control, Taxman has reported that drug offenders who are offered drug treatment services in prison have improved outcomes.[19] Treatment is associated with a reduced incidence of criminal behaviour and increases the crime-free duration period. Even despite its coercive nature, substance use treatment services in prison have better completion rates than voluntary treatment programmes. Treatment may even be perceived in a positive light. Individuals have the opportunity to use their prison term to receive care for their substance use dependence.[20]

Coordination and accountability are the key components in substance use treatment programmes in prison. A certain number of components are necessary when coordinating treatment between the medical and prison systems. These include:

➤ establishing smooth lines of communication between criminal justice and treatment providers
➤ providing a continuum of care for the offenders
➤ using drug testing to monitor performances
➤ developing and implementing policies and eventual sanctions to increase compliance with treatment.

Those attending community after-care have reduced substance use and a better economic outcome than those who do not.[21] Community-based follow-up must be prepared prior to release. One example of re-entry guidelines is the Kentucky Re-Entry Guidelines for Drug Abusing Offenders (USA).[22] The guidelines include six points:

1 Increased communication and collaboration among agencies to establish a continuum of care upon re-entry.

2   Consistency within and across prison-based and community-based treatment to increase treatment participation and decrease relapse upon re-entry.

3   Tailor-made re-entry to meet each inmate's needs. Transition to community-based care should begin at least six months prior to release to ensure that individual context and barriers are adequately addressed.

4   Adequate preparation and attention should be given to key areas such as housing, social security coverage, employment and family support to ensure smoother transition to community life.

5   Community support systems (Alcoholics Anonymous/Narcotics Anonymous) should be identified and attendance encouraged.

6   Adequate follow-up and support for progress in key areas should also be provided.

The guidelines focus on improving the overall situation of released prisoners and providing support and guidance for smoother transitions to community life. Treatment programmes should also be coordinated with other community-based providers. Many individuals are co-infected with HIV and hepatitis C. Contacts with community-based treatment providers should be established prior to release to ensure a smooth transition and continuity in care. Prison release and contacts with community care should be established between three and six months prior to release.

KEY POINT 14.5

- Substance-dependence treatment should be proposed to all individuals with a substance use problem.
- Treatment plans should be elaborated to meet individual needs.
- In-prison treatment should be articulated with community-based care prior to release to optimise care and follow-up.

SUICIDE IN PRISON

Suicide represents the third leading cause of death after natural causes and HIV infection in prison. Suicide rates (US) attain between 18 and 40 per 100 000.[23] Rates are significantly greater than in the general population. In the United States, suicide rates are eight times that of the general population; in the United Kingdom, rates are five times that of the general population. In addition, suicide rates remain high in this population after their release from prison.[24]

Several factors are specifically related to increased suicide risk in prison. Isolation, punitive sanctions, severely restricted living conditions, unexpected additional charges and severe sanctions were all associated with increased suicide risk.[23,24] Isolation, deprivation and severe punishment during imprisonment are often associated with increased suicide risks. These potentially cause increased levels of stress, depression and anxiety that lead to suicidal thoughts and acts. Hanging was by far the most commonly used method (85%), followed by laceration or phlebotomy (6%) and overdose (3%).[25,26] Box 14.3 indicates some prison suicide risk factors.[27]

BOX 14.3 Prison suicide risk factors[27]

Epidemiological
- Male
- White race
- Married.

Criminological
- Occupation of a single cell
- Detainee or remand
- Serving a life sentence.

Clinical factors
- Recent suicidal ideation
- Current psychiatric diagnosis
- Receiving psychotropic medication.

Concerning psychiatric disorders, the greatest suicide risks are observed among prisoners with bipolar disorder, major depressive disorder, schizophrenia and non-schizophrenic psychotic disorder (greatest risk).[28] There are very few studies of suicide prevention interventions. Efforts should be made to train prison personnel in sensitive sectors such as high security areas and isolation to recognise psychotic behaviour and signs of depression. Two valuable screening tools may be used in the prison setting: SCOPE and Suicide Potential Scale.[29] Highly vulnerable populations, such as individuals who have recently been condemned or who have recently received a severe sentence, should also benefit from psychological support, or at least careful surveillance during the period following their integration into the prison environment.

KEY POINT 14.6

Perhaps the greatest misconception is that talking about suicide incites suicidal acts. Suicidal thoughts are often present in prisoners. Lending an ear, offering support and appropriate referrals are on the contrary the first steps towards prevention.

The prison environment may be a source of excessive stress to individuals experiencing severe mentally illness. Judiciary policy efforts should be oriented towards more adapted means of incarcerating mentally ill offenders.[30] They should include:
➤ reinforced psychiatric care and follow-up
➤ a calm, community-oriented living situation with a small population.

These facilities should also provide services to support post-incarceration reinsertion and promote community-based psychiatric follow-up.

INDIVIDUALS WITH SPECIAL NEEDS: WOMEN

SELF-ASSESSMENT EXERCISE 14.1

- Can you name some of the conditions (socioeconomic, relations, family . . .) which can contribute to poor health and reduced psychological well-being in women?
- Can you think of any actions which could be particularly helpful to women and that could contribute to improving their well-being in prison?
- Which psychiatric diseases should be especially screened in women?

Incarcerated women should be of special concern to both medical and psychiatric physicians. Women are a minority group within the judiciary system. According to 2006 figures, almost 113 000 women were incarcerated in state and federal prisons in the United States (7% of the total prison population). Women represented 12.7% of the overall jail population in the United States.[31]

The offences committed by women are also very different from men. Women are more often imprisoned for drug offences (18%), or property-related offences (31%), such as petty theft, than men. Driving while intoxicated represented 17% of offences. Only 17% of all violent offences were committed by women.[31]

Imprisoned women are characterised by deficient socioeconomic and psychological resources, high rates of substance use and of lifetime victimisation (physical and sexual abuse). Their educational level is often low and they have often held poorly paying jobs with little job stability. Minorities (e.g. African American) comprise nearly half of the American prison population.[32,33]

Most women are also mothers (80%), most with custody of children under 18 years.[32,33] Loss of contact with their children and loss of custody are major concerns of these women and have a significant impact on their mental well-being.

Drug use and dependence rates range from 30%–60% among women entering prison, according to various studies.[34] In a recent study among female British inmates, heroin and crack were the most frequently used drugs among daily users (68.8% and 66.2%, respectively), followed by benzodiazepines and cannabis. More than one drug per day was used in 77.8% of the daily users. Excessive alcohol consumption was also frequently associated with drug use.[35]

Mental illness is highly prevalent among females. The prevalence of major depression was slightly greater (12%) and personality disorder slightly less (42%, with 21% antisocial) than in male prisoners.[1] Many women suffer from post-traumatic stress disorder (PTSD) due to physical and sexual abuse. One study found PTSD rates that were 6 to 10 times that of the general population.[36] These individuals are of significant concern since they also have high rates of mental health–substance use, such as major depression and substance use disorder. Suicide attempts are also a concern since almost 50% of all females have made at least one suicide attempt prior to imprisonment.[37]

These statistics suggest that women in prison have certain gender specific needs that must be addressed during incarceration. They also indicate a major need for drug treatment and mental healthcare programmes in women's prisons. However, women are a minority among the overall prison population. Women require person-centred programmes that take into account not only 'physical' needs, but also their social, educational and psychological needs. Programmes must integrate substance use treatment, interventions to develop coping strategies for post-trauma and abuse, mental and physical health services, educational and vocational training and social services to assist in community reinsertion.

INDIVIDUALS WITH SPECIAL NEEDS: JUVENILE OFFENDERS

SELF-ASSESSMENT EXERCISE 14.2

> * Why is juvenile mental health and drug use screening important?
> * What actions would be important to improve mental health–substance use screening and care during and after detention?

One of the greatest challenges to healthcare professionals in prison is the juvenile population. In line with US constitutional rights to humane treatment during detention, the National Commission on Correctional Health Care (NCCHC) guidelines recommend rapid screening for mental health–substance use disorders in all juveniles.[38] However, the few prevalence studies that exist have shown what a daunting task this represents. The Northwestern Juvenile Project has shown a significantly greater proportion of mental health–substance use disorders among juveniles than in the general population.[39] This study showed that nearly three of four young women and two of three young men suffer from either a mental health or a substance use disorder. Conduct disorders were frequent (about 40%), but rarely isolated from other disorders. Teenage girls had a significantly greater prevalence of affective disorders and major depressive episodes, anxiety disorders and panic disorders as well as substance use disorders, excluding alcohol and marijuana.[40] Other disorder prevalences (psychosis, conduct disorder) were similar to those in teenage boys.

Another significant challenge to meeting juvenile detainee needs is the rapid turnover. Juvenile detention centres are transitory structures designed to hold minors while awaiting trial or before they are moved to a more permanent structure. Although an investment in a long-term care plan is not feasible, an initial positive contact, followed by a referral to an appropriate community or prison-based structure, would be ideal for those with less serious illness.

Which youths require immediate treatment? As for adults, it is important that any current treatments (opiate substitution, psychiatrist prescriptions) be continued during detention. It is also important that any major depressive disorders, manic disorders and acute withdrawal syndromes be seen and rapidly managed by a psychiatrist.

Screening for suicidal ideation and conduct is another important part of juvenile health interviewing. Suicidal ideation is very frequent among adolescents. It is also common in juvenile detainees (nearly half).[41,42] For many, this initial mental health screen is the first time they are able to verbalise their suicidal thoughts and an important step towards prevention. In practice, it is important to simply and directly ask the individual if he/she has thought about suicide in the last three months. An individual who expresses suicidal thoughts or has a history of skin cuttings, auto-mutilations or suicide attempts should be referred to a psychiatrist for further evaluation.

Although these individuals present significant challenges in terms of volume and rapid response, many advocates believe it is also an excellent opportunity for prevention of future incarcerations and the establishment of a mental healthcare plan. These actions could also carry the long-term benefits of improved socio-professional integration and improved well-being for troubled individuals.

CONCLUSION

Mental health–substance use problems are commonplace among prisoners. Thus, the needs for effective mental health screening and targeted psychiatric referrals in prisons, jails and detention centres are significant. The need for appropriate social and psychiatric support to special groups, such as women and youth, is also essential and severely lacking in today's prison system. Despite proofs of their efficacy, the means provided to mental health professionals in prisons are largely inadequate. It could be hoped that future prison policies will integrate improvements in healthcare to this needy population.

REFERENCES

1 Fazel S, Danesh J. Serious mental disorder in 23 000 prisoners: a systematic review of 62 surveys. *Lancet.* 2002; **359**: 545–50.

2 Lamb HR, Weinberger LE, Marsh JS, *et al.* Treatment prospects for persons with severe mental illness in an urban county jail. *Psychiatric Services.* 2007; **58**: 782–6.

3 James D, Glaze L. *Mental Health Problems of Prison and Jail Inmates.* Rockville, MD: US Department of Justice; 2006.

4 Greenberg GA, Rosenheck RA. Jail incarceration, homelessness, and mental health: a national study. *Psychiatric Services.* 2008; **59**: 170–7.

5 Blitz CL, Wolff N, Shi J. Physical victimization in prison: the role of mental illness. *International Journal of Law Psychiatry.* 2008; **31**: 385–93.

6 Teplin LA, McClelland GM, Abram KM, *et al.* Crime victimization in adults with severe mental illness: comparison with the National Crime Victimization Survey. *Archives of General Psychiatry.* 2005; **62**: 911–21.

7 Yang S, Kadouri A, Revah-Levy A, *et al.* Doing time: a qualitative study of long-term incarceration and the impact of mental illness. *International Journal of Law Psychiatry.* 2009; **32**: 294–303.

8 World Health Organization. *Health in Prisons Project Group. Background Paper for Trenčín Statement on Prisons and Mental Health.* Copenhagen: World Health Organization Regional Office for Europe; 2008.

9 Steadman HJ, Scott JE, Osher F, *et al.* Validation of the brief jail mental health screen. *Psychiatric Services.* 2005; **56**: 816–22.

10 Veysey BM, Steadman HJ, Morrissey JP, *et al.* Using the Referral Decision Scale to screen mentally ill jail detainees: validity and implementation issues. *Law and Human Behavior.* 1998; **22**: 205–15.

11 White P, Chant D. The psychometric properties of a psychosis screen in a correctional setting. *International Journal of Law Psychiatry.* 2006; **29**: 137–44.

12 Peters RH, Greenbaum PE, Steinberg ML, *et al.* Effectiveness of screening instruments in detecting substance use disorders among prisoners. *Journal of Substance Abuse Treatment.* 2000; **18**: 349–58.

13 Simpson D, Knight K. *TCU Data Collection Forms for Correctional Residential Treatment.* Fort Worth, TX: Texas Christian University; 1998.

14 Saxon AJ, Kivlahan DR, Doyle S, *et al.* Further validation of the alcohol dependence scale as an index of severity. *Journal of Studies on Alcohol Drugs.* 2007; **68**: 149–56.

15 Gordon MS, Kinlock TW, Schwartz RP, *et al.* A randomized clinical trial of methadone maintenance for prisoners: findings at 6 months post-release. *Addiction.* 2008; **103**: 1333–42.

16 Kinlock TW, Gordon MS, Schwartz RP, *et al.* A study of methadone maintenance for male prisoners: 3-month postrelease outcomes. *Criminal Justice and Behavior.* 2008; **35**: 34–47.

17 Benyamina A, Blecha L, Lebeau B, Reynaud M. Prevention of HIV transmission among intravenous drug users. *Lancet.* 2010; **375**: 1782.

18 Mathers BM, Degenhardt L, Ali H, *et al.* HIV prevention, treatment, and care services for people who inject drugs: a systematic review of global, regional, and national coverage. *Lancet.* 2010; **375**: 1014–28.

19 Taxman FS, Perdoni ML, Harrison LD. Drug treatment services for adult offenders: the state of the state. *Journal of Substance Abuse Treatment.* 2007; **32**: 239–54.

20 Stewart D. Drug use and perceived treatment need among newly sentenced prisoners in England and Wales. *Addiction.* 2009; **104**: 243–7.

21 O'Connell DJ, Enev TN, Martin SS, *et al.* Working toward recovery: the interplay of past treatment and economic status in long-term outcomes for drug-involved offenders. *Substance Use and Misuse.* 2007; **42**: 1089–107.

22 Stanton-Tindall M, Rees J, Oser C, *et al.* Establishing partnerships between correctional agencies and university researchers to enhance substance abuse treatment initiatives. *Corrections Today.* 2007; **69**: 42–5.

23 Daniel AE. Preventing suicide in prison: a collaborative responsibility of administrative, custodial, and clinical staff. *Journal of the American Academy Psychiatry Law.* 2006; **34**: 165–75.

24 Fazel S, Benning R, Danesh J. Suicides in male prisoners in England and Wales, 1978–2003. *Lancet.* 2005; **366**: 1301–2.

25 Dooley E. Prison suicide in England and Wales, 1972–87. *British Journal of Psychiatry.* 1990; **156**: 40–5.

26 Shaw J, Baker D, Hunt IM, *et al.* Suicide by prisoners. National clinical survey. *British Journal of Psychiatry.* 2004; **184**: 263–7.

27 Fazel S, Cartwright J, Norman-Nott A, *et al.* Suicide in prisoners: a systematic review of risk factors. *Journal of Clinical Psychiatry.* 2008; **69**: 1721–31.

28 Baillargeon J, Penn JV, Thomas CR, *et al.* Psychiatric disorders and suicide in the nation's largest state prison system. *Journal of the American Academy of Psychiatry Law.* 2009; **37**: 188–93.

29 Perry AE, Marandos R, Coulton S, *et al.* Screening tools assessing risk of suicide and self-harm in adult offenders: a systematic review. *International Journal of Offender Therapy and Comparative Criminology.* 2010; **54**(5): 803–28. 11 March Epub/2010. doi: 10.1177/0306624X09359757.

30 Konrad N, Daigle MS, Daniel AE, *et al.* Preventing suicide in prisons, part I. Recommendations

from the International Association for Suicide Prevention Task Force on Suicide in Prisons. *Crisis*. 2007; **28**: 113–21.

31 Sabol W, Couture H, Harrison P. *Prisoners in 2006*. Washington, DC: Bureau of Justice Statistics Bulletin, NCJ 219416; 2007.

32 Bloom BE, Owen BA, Covington S, National Institute of Corrections (US). *Gender-responsive Strategies: research, practice, and guiding principles for women offenders*. Washington, DC: US Department of Justice, National Institute of Corrections; 2003.

33 Gunter TD. Incarcerated women and depression: a primer for the primary care provider. *Journal of American Medical Women's Association*. 2004; **59**: 107–12.

34 Moloney KP, Moller LF. Good practice for mental health programming for women in prison: reframing the parameters. *Public Health*. 2009; **123**: 431–3.

35 Plugge E, Yudkin P, Douglas N. Changes in women's use of illicit drugs following imprisonment. *Addiction*. 2009; **104**: 215–22.

36 Goff A, Rose E, Rose S, *et al*. Does PTSD occur in sentenced prison populations? A systematic literature review. *Criminal Behaviour and Mental Health*. 2007; **17**: 152–62.

37 Borrill J, Burnett R, Atkins R, *et al*. Patterns of self-harm and attempted suicide among white and black/mixed race female prisoners. *Criminal Behaviour and Mental Health*. 2003; **13**: 229–40.

38 Wasserman GA, Jensen PS, Ko SJ, *et al*. Mental health assessments in juvenile justice: report on the consensus conference. *Journal of the American Academy of Child and Adolescent Psychiatry*. 2003; **42**: 752–61.

39 Teplin LA, Abram KM, McClelland GM, *et al*. Detecting mental disorder in juvenile detainees: who receives services. *American Journal of Public Health*. 2005; **95**: 1773–80.

40 Teplin LA, Abram KM, McClelland GM, *et al*. Psychiatric disorders in youth in juvenile detention. *Archives of General Psychiatry*. 2002; **59**: 1133–43.

41 Hayes LM. Juvenile suicide in confinement in the United States results from a national survey. *Crisis*. 2005; **26**: 146–8.

42 Roberts AR, Bender K. Juvenile offender suicide: prevalence, risk factors, assessment, and crisis intervention protocols. *International Journal of Emergency Mental Health*. 2006; **8**: 255–65.

TO LEARN MORE

- Center for Gender and Justice: www.centerforgenderandjustice.org
- King's College London International Centre for Prison Studies: www.kcl.ac.uk/schools/law/research/icps
- National Institute of Corrections: http://nicic.gov
- Centre for Mental Health: www.scmh.org.uk
- US Department of Justice, Office of Justice Programs: www.ojp.usdoj.gov
- Young Minds Stressed Out and Struggling (SOS) Project: www.youngminds.org/
- Moller L, Stöver H, Jürgens R, *et al*. editors. *Health in Prisons: a WHO guide to the essentails in prison health*. World Health Organization; 2007. www.asca.net/documents/e90174-Health InPris.pdf
- Office of Juvenile Justice and Delinquency Prevention, US Department of Justice Office of Justice Programs: Information concerning the Northwestern Juvenile Project. Available at: www.ncjrs.gov/pdffiles1/ojjdp/fs200102.pdf
- Training Institute for Suicide Assessment: www.suicideassessment.com

CHAPTER 15

Communicating harm reduction

Cheryl Kipping

This chapter commences with an overview of harm reduction before considering when and how to deliver harm reduction interventions. Suggestions on how harm reduction can be made part of routine practice are made before resources that may be helpful in supporting such work are identified.

INTRODUCTION

Substance use (alcohol, licit or illicit drugs and tobacco) can have harmful consequences for anyone. For people with mental health problems these can be particularly severe and even a low level of substance use, that would not usually be considered harmful in people without mental health problems, can have a significant impact. Harms may concern the person's mental health, physical health, social situation (relationships, ability to care for children or dependent relatives, finances, housing/accommodation, and education/employment) and legal situation. Despite this, like many others in society, people with mental health problems continue to use substances. Harm reduction acknowledges that, although abstinence from substances would be desirable, some people will continue to use them, so finding ways of reducing the associated harms is a pragmatic way forward.

Harm reduction has been defined as policies, programmes, services and actions to reduce health, social and economic harms to individuals, communities, and societies.[1] It derives from the drugs field, where there has been an emphasis on reducing the harms associated with intravenous drug use. For example, needle exchange schemes have been introduced to reduce the transmission of blood-borne viruses. The harm-reduction/minimisation (the terms harm reduction and harm minimisation tend to be used interchangeably) approach can, however, be applied to any substance. Responding to concerns about the individual, community and societal harms associated with drug and alcohol use, the UK government has made reducing these a priority.[2]

Harms associated with mental illness tend to be thought of in terms of risk. Regardless of whether the focus is on mental health or substance use the principles of risk management/harm reduction are similar. For people with mental health–substance use problems harm reduction is a first step in care and treatment.[3,4]

Harm reduction is underpinned by health education: providing information so that people can make informed choices about their behaviour and lifestyle.

Providing health education information is, then, an important component of harm reduction.

SELF-ASSESSMENT EXERCISE 15.1

Time: 15 minutes
Read this case study then identify possible health, social and economic harms at the individual, community and societal levels.

Rob is a 37-year-old married man with two children aged five and three. Five years ago his brother was killed in a car accident. Rob had been driving the car. He blamed himself. Soon after his brother's death Rob started drinking alcohol heavily to help him cope with his feelings of guilt and loss. Over time his drinking escalated and he became physically dependent. He started taking time off work and, although initially his employer was supportive, eventually Rob lost his job. To ensure that the family could meet their financial commitments, his wife, Jane, took on extra work. Rob has experienced extended periods of low mood and, at times, has felt suicidal. On one occasion, he was picked up by the police near a railway line and admitted to a psychiatric ward because of concerns about his suicide risk. During the admission, he was detoxified from alcohol. Having been informed that his blood tests showed signs of liver damage, and recognising the impact that alcohol was having on his life and that of his family, Rob engaged with local alcohol services. After a few months, he dropped out of treatment and began drinking again. His relationship with his wife has become increasingly difficult. They have frequent arguments and the ongoing demands of their situation are taking their toll on her. Her physical and mental health is deteriorating. Concerns have also emerged in relation to their children. Sometimes Rob looks after them until Jane returns from work. On one occasion, he left the children at home while he went to the shop. One of them left the house and was found in the street by a community police officer. A referral to children and families social services was made.

DELIVERING HARM REDUCTION INTERVENTIONS

This section begins by identifying key elements that underpin delivery of harm reduction interventions. It then identifies when harm reduction is appropriate and considers what interventions might be delivered. The focus is on working with people in contact with mental health services.

Key elements underpinning delivery of harm reduction interventions
Working in partnership
A positive relationship between the individual and professional is an important prerequisite for the delivery of harm reduction interventions. Establishing a relationship can, in itself, be a challenge. Some people are reluctant to engage with mental health services yet they can be the people experiencing the most harm. Professionals need to work imaginatively and flexibly to create opportunities for developing positive therapeutic relationships (*see* Book 4, Chapter 2).

Once established, a partnership approach is required through which the individual is supported to make life choices. Professionals need to be empathic, non-judgemental, respectful of choices (even when they do not agree with them), and believe that changes are possible (therapeutic optimism).[5] This contrasts with the confrontational approach sometimes taken by professionals. People who use services are told that substance use is bad for them and that they should stop. Such an approach is likely to create tensions in the relationship resulting in a reluctance to discuss use in an open way and closing off opportunities for constructive dialogue about change. While abstinence is the ultimate harm reduction goal, pushing for it when the person does not want, or is unable, to stop use is not in keeping with the harm reduction approach.

REFLECTIVE PRACTICE EXERCISE 15.1

Time: 15 minutes
- Some people think that harm reduction condones, and even encourages, substance use. What do you think?
- Is it an appropriate approach for professionals to take, or should abstinence be advocated?

Integrated treatment model

Mental health and substance use problems cannot be seen in isolation; each is likely to impact on the other. An integrated treatment model, where both are addressed at the same time, in one setting, by one team, is therefore the most appropriate.[3] Understanding the interrelationships between mental health, substance use and other aspects of a person's life will be important if achievable harm reduction plans are to be devised.

Professional knowledge about substances and how harms can be reduced

For professionals to provide health education/harm reduction information they need a good understanding of the substances that may be used, their methods of use and the adverse effects each may have. A good understanding of the risks associated with mental illness is also required, as well as the ways in which substances can exacerbate mental health risks. Building on this knowledge, an awareness of the steps that might be taken to reduce harms is required.

Tables 15.1 and 15.2 provide information about some of the health harms associated with mental health–substance use. Table 15.1 focuses on routes of drug administration and includes suggestions on how the identified harms can be addressed. Table 15.2 identifies health harms associated with alcohol, cannabis and stimulant drugs (particularly crack cocaine). These are the substances most commonly used by people with mental health problems. The information provided is not exhaustive; it does, however, provide readers with some insights that can be drawn upon to inform practice.

TABLE 15.1 Harms associated with routes of administration

Injecting		Smoking/inhaling	
Harms	**Methods of reducing harms**	**Harms**	**Methods of reducing harms**
• Transmission of blood-borne viruses (hepatitis B, C, HIV)	• Stop injecting, change route to, e.g. skin-pop or smoke	• Hot smoke can cause bronchial damage	• Water pipes can cool smoke and filter out some contaminants
• Local infections, e.g. abscesses	• Hepatitis A and B vaccination	• Inhaling can precipitate asthma and other respiratory problems	• Use screen/gauze in pipe/bong to reduce amount of ash/embers inhaled
• Systemic infections, e.g. septicaemia, endocarditis	• Test for hepatitis C and HIV and treat accordingly	• Mixing with tobacco will result in tobacco-related harms	• Eat or make tea
• Vein/artery damage – also acids used to prepare substances for injection can cause vein damage – reusing needles increases risk of vein damage	• Use clean injecting equipment (spoons, filters, water, needles, syringes); and dispose of safely	• Nasal inhalation, snorting, sniffing (e.g. powdered cocaine, amphetamine) can cause breathing problems and atrophy of nasal septum	• Avoid inhaling too deeply or holding smoke for too long
• Deep vein thrombosis	• If reusing equipment ensure know most effective way of cleaning it		• Always use own pipe
• Accidental overdose	• If using with others mark/label own equipment to reduce risk of sharing	• Specific risks may be associated with the materials used to make pipes, e.g. fumes given off by plastic bottles or from paint on aluminium tins can be inhaled	• Clean smoking equipment regularly
• Injecting into groin (artery and nerve nearby), neck (artery nearby)	• Wash hands and clean surfaces on which injection being prepared		• Drink water to help keep hydrated and prevent lips cracking
• Poor general health	• Education regarding overdose risk, e.g. tolerance/loss of tolerance, awareness of varying purity, do not mix with other CNS depressants, do not inject	• Risk of blood-borne virus transmission as result of cuts from tin cans or burns around mouth	• Use lip balm
Crack cocaine specific:			• Ensure registered with general practitioner so that health needs can be addressed
• Anaesthetic effect reduces awareness of damage at injecting sites			

(continued)

TABLE 15.1 (*cont.*)

Injecting		Smoking/inhaling	
Harms	**Methods of reducing harms**	**Harms**	**Methods of reducing harms**
• Increases risk of seizures, strokes, heart attack • If speedballing (injection of heroin with crack/cocaine) can lose track of amount of heroin used and increase risk of overdose.	• Use with others, not alone • Safer injecting advice (rotate injection sites, use smallest needle/bore possible, avoid neck, groin, breast, penis, feet, hands) • Take care of general healthcare • Ensure tetanus immunisation up to date • First aid training, e.g. management of unconscious person for service users, family and friends • Ensure registered with GP so that health needs can be addressed ***Opiate specific:*** • Substitute prescribing (e.g. methadone, buprenorphine) • Naloxone (to be administered by friends/family in case of overdose).	• Risk of spreading bacterial infections by sharing joints, bongs.	

TABLE 15.2 Harms associated with specific substances

Substance	Alcohol	Cannabis	Stimulants
Physical health	• Accidents due to impaired coordination and/or judgement • Interactions with other substances/medication • Cognitive impairment • Withdrawal seizures • Delirium tremens • Wernicke's encephalopathy • Peripheral neuritis • Link to range of physical diseases, liver cirrhosis, gastrointestinal disorders, heart disease, pancreatitis, skin problems, cancers, etc. • Overdose • Inhalation of vomit • Disruption of sleep patterns • Falls when intoxicated	• Damage to respiratory system • Impaired cognitive functioning • Impaired coordination • Accidents due to impaired coordination and/or judgement	• Respiratory problems (wheezing, shortness of breath, 'crack lung') • Cardiovascular problems (raised blood pressure, arrthymias, strokes, heart attack) • Seizures (associated with overheating/raised body temperature) • Prolonged use can lead to poor general health due to lack of sleep, food
Mental health	• Can induce/exacerbate anxiety, depression • Can induce alcoholic hallucinosis • Reduces inhibitions, increasing likelihood of acts of self-harm, suicide and violence.	• Can precipitate agitation, anxiety, suspiciousness • Can trigger/exacerbate psychosis • Can trigger/exacerbate depression.	• May trigger/exacerbate psychosis • Depression associated with withdrawal/comedown – this can increase risk of suicide • Anxiety, agitation, irritability, restlessness.

Comprehensive assessment

A detailed understanding of the individual, his/her circumstances and the role that substances play in his/her life is required if effective harm reduction interventions are to be delivered. A comprehensive bio-psychosocial assessment is therefore needed. This will reveal risks/harms and may provide pointers to ways in which these could be addressed. Key information required to shape harm reduction interventions is highlighted below.

SUBSTANCE USE

Essential information includes:

➤ what substances the person is taking
➤ how much the person is using
➤ how frequently the use is
➤ the route of, and practice in relation to, use/administration
➤ how long the person has been using substances at the current level
➤ the circumstances in which the person uses substances (e.g. alone/with others, at home/in a 'crack house')
➤ patterns of substance use (e.g. consistent/stable or chaotic, using one substance to counter effect of another)
➤ withdrawal symptoms
➤ experience of overdoses (accidental or deliberate).

MENTAL HEALTH

As well as gaining information about current and past mental health problems, and the factors that may precipitate or protect against these, constructing a chronological timeline that brings together information about significant life events, mental health and substance use may provide insights into the relationship between substance use and mental health.

PHYSICAL HEALTH

Harms to physical health may be acute or chronic. Given the very significant health problems that can be associated with mental health–substance use, a thorough assessment of current and past health is required along with physical examination and other relevant tests. Attention also needs to be given to sexual health; some people will be involved in sex work to support their substance use.

MEDICATION

Details of all prescribed medications are required, as well as information about whether these are being taken as prescribed. The potentially dangerous interactions between prescribed medication and other substances need to be considered.

SOCIAL SITUATION

An understanding of the person's social circumstances is required:

➤ relationships
➤ ability to care for children or dependent adults
➤ accommodation
➤ education/employment
➤ finances; including how they are financing their substance use and any debts (particularly to dealers).

LEGAL ISSUES

If the person is using illicit substances they will be involved in illegal activity because of their use. Some people may engage in criminal activity to fund use; others may be involved in illegal activity as a consequence of use (e.g. drink-driving). Details of criminal activity and any convictions/sentences should be obtained.

RISK ASSESSMENT

This should bring together information gained from the other assessment domains and identify any additional risks, such as:

➤ accidents
➤ self-neglect
➤ abuse/exploitation/vulnerability.

REASONS FOR USE, PERCEPTION OF WHETHER (OR NOT) USE IS A PROBLEM AND READINESS TO CHANGE

Gaining a sense of how the individual views use, the role substance use plays in his/her life and whether or not use is seem as problematic is important for negotiating goals and care planning.

Identifying when harm reduction is appropriate

Using the 'cycle of change' model[6] (*see* Figure 15.1; and also Book 4, Chapter 6) as a framework, and drawing on the assessment information, the professional can identify when harm reduction is likely to be appropriate. The cycle of change model sees change as a process where the person moves from precontemplation, where their behaviour/lifestyle is not seen as problematic and significant change is therefore not considered, through to contemplation, where there is some acknowledgement of difficulties and the possibility of change is considered, on to preparation/determination where plans for change are made, and then action, when change is made.

Harm reduction interventions are generally targeted at people at the precontemplation and contemplation stages. In the former, the emphasis is likely to be on addressing practical issues, such as ensuring the person has adequate accommodation and food. At the contemplation stage, because people have at least partially acknowledged the harmful consequences associated with their mental health–substance use, more collaborative discussion can take place about the possibility of change to reduce these harms.

Identifying appropriate harm reduction interventions

Once an understanding has been gained of the harms the person is experiencing and it has been established that she/he does not want, or feels unable, to stop using substances, Maslow's hierarchy of needs is a helpful model for identifying harm reduction goals (*see* Figure 15.2).[7] Maslow suggests that needs at the lower levels must be met before those higher up can be addressed. Initial harm reduction interventions, then, are likely to relate to physiological and safety needs.

Safety needs relating to security and protection may also need to be prioritised, particularly if the person is at risk of seriously harming her- or himself or others because of a disturbed mental state and/or chaotic substance using lifestyle. The professional has a responsibility to protect the individual, and others, and may need to act in ways that are contrary to the individual's wishes, for example arranging a

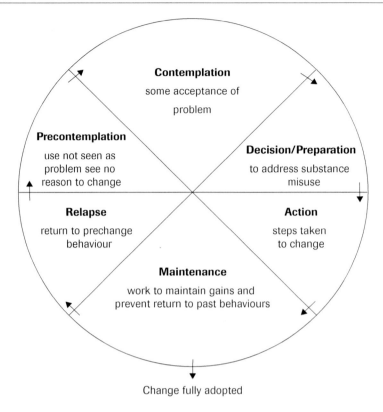

FIGURE 15.1 The cycle of change[6]

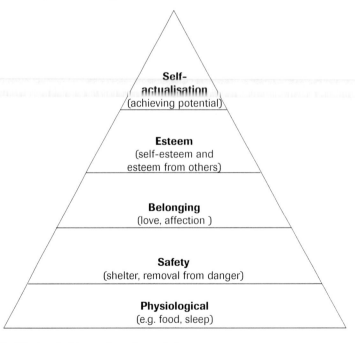

FIGURE 15.2 Maslow's hierarchy of needs[7]

mental health assessment that may result in enforced hospitalisation.

Once the person's basic needs have been met, and some stability has been achieved, it will be possible to work in a more collaborative way on the individual's concerns. This may include discussing crises so that an advanced care plan can be negotiated to guide management of similar circumstances should they arise in the future.

Although the individual will probably be aware of some the negative impacts the mental health–substance use is having, she/he may be unaware of others, particularly those that are not immediately obvious. A key aspect of the professionals' role is to make information available about potential harms, and ways in which these might be reduced, so that the individual can make informed choices about her/his behaviour. Part of this process will be eliciting the person's current knowledge about substances and the impact they may be having so that the information provided can be modified to meet the particular individual's needs. Another aspect may be discussing the relative advantages and disadvantages of potential courses of action, particularly when reducing harm in one area may elevate it in another. For example, to reduce the harms to the respiratory system associated with smoking cannabis the individual might decide to eat it (in cakes). This method of consumption, however, reduces the person's ability to control its intoxicating effects. If the person started feeling anxious and suspicious and she/he was smoking a 'joint', these feelings might be moderated by reducing the frequency of inhaling, or stopping use at that time. If the cannabis has been eaten, it is already in the person's body and there is no way of moderating its effects, which may last several hours.

Motivational interviewing[8] is an essential skill, particularly at this stage. The change goals, which may be in one or more domains (physical or mental health, social or legal), and decisions about the strategies for achieving them, must be those of the individual. It is important for goals to be realistic. Achieving small goals can build confidence and self-esteem and encourage further changes. Failing to achieve ambitious goals can result in a sense of hopelessness and failure. So, for example, a realistic goal for a heavy drinker who usually starts drinking at midday might be to wait until 1 p.m., rather than, say, 5 p.m. Over time, the more ambitious goal may be achieved through small, incremental steps. The goals identified by the individual and plans for how these will be achieved should be set out in a care plan. Regular review with the individual is important so that progress is evaluated. A successful outcome is achieved if the individual attains the harm reduction goal.

Addressing the needs of families/carers

As highlighted in the case of Rob (Self-assessment exercise 15.1), family and carers may experience harm as a consequence of the mental health–substance use of others. Professionals have a responsibility to consider the needs of family and carers. Family and/or carers' assessments provide an opportunity to do this. Some direct intervention with the family may be appropriate, for example:

➤ making a referral to children and families social services if there are concerns about child welfare
➤ providing written and verbal information about substance use, mental health and the interrelationships between them

➤ providing advice on how to access help in emergency situations
➤ providing training on managing the harms the individual is experiencing (e.g. first aid; *see* Book 3, Chapter 9 – administering naloxone)
➤ providing information about family/carer support groups.

SELF-ASSESSMENT EXERCISE 15.2

Time: 60 minutes

Natalie is a 30-year-old black British woman who has a diagnosis of schizophrenia. She is on depot medication, which controls her symptoms well. She also has a substance use problem. Her drug of choice is crack cocaine, which she uses on a regular basis (most days). She also drinks alcohol most days, typically two cans of strong cider, and will use other substances if they are offered to her, e.g. cannabis and heroin. On occasions, she has used heroin intravenously. To fund her use Natalie borrows money from family and friends, she shoplifts and engages in sex for money and/or drugs. She has a long list of convictions and has served a custodial sentence for theft (snatched a handbag). Natalie has two children who live with her mother. She can have supervised access. At times when her substance use escalates, she tends to neglect herself. She also becomes more difficult to engage with mental health services, missing appointments, not staying at her flat and not answering her phone.

● What harms might Natalie experience because of her mental health–substance use? Consider harm in relation to physical and mental health, and social and legal circumstances.
● Identify how services might work with Natalie to reduce these harms. Devise a possible care plan.
● Think of an individual with whom you are working. What harms does she/he experience because of mental health–substance use? Consider harm in relation to physical and mental health, and social and legal circumstances.
● Identify how you might work with this person to reduce the harms. Devise a possible care plan. Remember that in reality care plans need to be developed collaboratively with the individual and focus on her/his goals.

MAKING HARM REDUCTION PART OF ROUTINE PRACTICE

Given the high prevalence of mental health–substance use and the fact that many people are unwilling or unable to stop using, harm reduction should be part of routine practice. This section provides some suggestions on how this might be achieved.

➤ Ensure that the risks/harms associated with substance use are identified in risk assessments, and a risk management/harm reduction care plan is devised:
— including prompts related to substance use, harms in risk assessment documentation may help professionals identify harms more consistently
— conducting audits can promote quality improvement.
➤ Ensure training is available to equip professionals with the capabilities required to deliver harm reduction interventions:

— could someone from the substance use team provide such training?
➤ Effectively utilising health promotion/harm reduction information resources:
  — posters and leaflets can be displayed in waiting rooms and communal areas of wards/residential settings
  — materials can be used in more structured work, such as individual and group sessions, and in professional training
  — if computer terminals with Internet access are available, websites that provide health education information and harm reduction advice can be saved as 'favourites' to make them easily accessible
  — nominate someone to be responsible for identifying appropriate resources for your clinical area and ensuring that stocks are maintained.
➤ Ensure information about local substance use services is available:
  — have some professionals that have visited the services and can talk knowledgeably about them
  — find out about these services' harm reduction resources and any initiatives your team could draw upon.
➤ Seek the views of the individual, family and carers on how harm reduction can be incorporated into services:
  — peer support/education might be an option.
➤ Have policies and procedures in place to:
  — minimise the use of substances on premises and manage the situation when it does occur
  — manage emergency situations, such as accidental overdose
  — disseminate widely 'alert' information, e.g. regarding contaminated heroin.
➤ Link harm reduction to other initiatives:
  — physical healthcare/healthy living groups
  — social inclusion activities, such as walking, gardening, sport
  — protected engagement time.
➤ Have a champion (e.g. substance use professional/physical healthcare lead/the individual), to promote harm reduction work.
➤ Work collaboratively and regularly share information with partner agencies and families/carers if agreed by the individual with mental health–substance use.
  — clarify confidentiality arrangements and seek consent for information sharing with the individual
  — ensure partner agencies and families/carers are invited to Care Programme Approach meetings and receive copies of care plans.
➤ Improve your practice by learning lessons from serious untoward incident investigations.

CONCLUSION

Although abstinence is the ultimate harm reduction goal and would often be professionals' preferred option for people experiencing mental health–substance use problems, the perceived benefits of substance use for many people result in them being unwilling or unable to stop. Harm reduction provides a pragmatic approach that aims to minimise harm to the person themselves, those with whom they have contact and wider society. Although some people will continue to use substances for many years, skilful delivery of harm reduction interventions can provide the foundation for longer-term, more significant change as the individual utilises the collaborative relationship established with the professional, recognises the benefits associated with achieving small changes, and builds on the greater sense of self-efficacy and confidence gained.

REFERENCES

1 United Kingdom Harm Reduction Alliance. Harm reduction defined; 2007. Available at: www.ukhra.org/harm_reduction_definition.html (accessed 18 May 2010).
2 Her Majesties Treasury. *PSA Delivery Agreement 25: reduce the harm caused by alcohol and drugs.* HMSO; 2009. Available at: www.hm-treasury.gov.uk/d/pbr_csr07_psa25.pdf (accessed 18 May 2010).
3 Department of Health. *Mental Health Policy Implementation Guide: dual diagnosis good practice guide.* London: Department of Health; 2002.
4 Department of Health. *Dual Diagnosis in Mental Health Inpatient and Day Hospital Settings.* London: Department of Health; 2006.
5 Hughes L. *Closing the Gap: a capability framework for working effectively with combined mental health and substance misuse problems (dual diagnosis).* Centre for Clinical and Workforce Innovation, University of Lincoln, Mansfield; 2006. Available at: www.lincoln. ac.uk/ccawi/publications/Closing%20the%20Gap.pdf (accessed 18 May 2010).
6 Prochaska JO, DiClemente CC. Towards a comprehensive model of change. In: Miller W, Heather N, editors. *Treating Addictive Behaviours: processes of change.* New York: Plenum; 1986.
7 Maslow AH. A theory of human motivation. *Psychological Review.* 1943; **50**: 370–96.
8 Miller W, Rollnick S, editors. *Motivational Interviewing: preparing people for change.* New York: Guilford Press; 2002.

TO LEARN MORE

A range of resources is available to support delivery of harm reduction. This section provides links to websites and identifies further reading that may be helpful.

Alcohol

- This site provides information about alcohol including the health harms and tips on reducing use. There is also an interactive element so that people can assess whether they are drinking too much: www.drinking.nhs.uk/questions/alcohol-units/
- The UK Department of Health produce a range of products (e.g. posters, unit calculators and booklets), aimed at raising awareness of safe drinking levels and the potentially harmful effects of alcohol. Some are targeted at healthcare professionals; others are for the general public. These resources are free. www.orderline.dh.gov.uk/ecom_dh/public/home.jsf;jsessionid=698 1E1466921E33BDF45AF6ABCD57EB5.plukweb1
- The Drinkaware Trust site contains information about alcohol and its effects. There is an interactive section and free resources, including fact sheets and unit calculators: www.drinkaware. co.uk
- Alcohol Concern produces fact sheets that can be downloaded for free: www.alcoholconcern. org.uk/
- For more in-depth information about working with people with drinking problems: Cooper

DB, editor. *Alcohol Use*. Oxford: Radcliffe Publishing; 2000; and Edwards G, Marshall EJ, Cook C. *The Treatment of Drinking Problems*. Cambridge: Cambridge University Press; 2003.

Drugs

- The FRANK website has lots of information about drugs and their effects. It also includes an interactive, self-help element. A range of free resources can also be ordered. Only small numbers can be ordered directly from the site: www.talktofrank.com. Larger quantities can be obtained by contacting: 0800 776600; or the UK Department of Health orderline: 0300 123 1002.
- The Lifeline provides lots of useful information about drugs and alcohol. Lifeline also produces excellent resources. There is a cost for these: www.lifelineproject.co.uk and www.lifeline publications.org. Of particular relevance to taking a harm reduction approach when working with people with mental health–substance use problems is the *Out of Your Head* guides.
- HIT provides a wide range of resources on drugs and alcohol. There is a charge for these products. *Crack Cocaine: reduce the risks* describes steps people can take to reduce the harm associated with use: www.hit.org.uk
- The Royal College of Psychiatrists site has information about alcohol and cannabis and mental health: www.rcpsych.ac.uk
- Know Cannabis provides information and has an interactive self-help element for people who are considering cutting down. Free information booklets are available. www.knowcannabis. org.uk
- The Harm Reduction Works website provides information targeted at injecting drug users so covers topics such as HIV, hepatitis B and C, safer injecting practice, and overdose prevention. As well as information on the site itself, materials can be ordered: posters, DVDs and booklets. They are free in England. www.harmreductionworks.org.uk
- Exchange Supplies provides information and products aimed at reducing the harms associated with injecting drug use. There is a charge for the resources. www.exchangesupplies.org

Useful chapters

The *Mental Health–Substance Use* series comprises six books. To develop knowledge and understanding, chapters are interlinked, building and exploring specific areas. It is hoped the following will help readers locate relevant chapters easily.

BOOK 1: INTRODUCTION TO MENTAL HEALTH–SUBSTANCE USE

1 Setting the scene
2 Learning to learn
3 What is in a name? The search for appropriate and consistent terminology
4 The mental health–substance use journey
5 A matter of human rights: people's right to healthcare for mental health–substance use
6 The importance of physical health assessment
7 The experience of illness
8 The psychological impact of serious illness
9 Working with people with mental health–substance use
10 Skills, capabilities and professional development: a response framework for mental health–substance use
11 Attitudes and brief training interventions: a practical approach
12 Ethics, mental health–substance use
13 Brain injury, mental health–substance use
14 Heatwave, mental health–substance use

BOOK 2: DEVELOPING SERVICES IN MENTAL HEALTH–SUBSTANCE USE

1 Setting the scene
2 Historical policy context of mental health–substance use
3 Epidemiological issues in mental health–substance use: a case for a life course approach to chronic disease epidemiology
4 National Mental Health Development Unit: an English perspective
5 Severe mental health and substance use: developing integrated services – a UK perspective
6 An Australian rural service system's journey towards systemic mental health–substance use capability
7 Developing and evaluating innovative community programmes
8 Guidelines for working with mental health–substance use

BOOK 6: PRACTICE IN MENTAL HEALTH–SUBSTANCE USE

Useful contacts

Collated by Jo Cooper

Addiction Arena – www.addictionarena.com

Addiction Medicine List – http://listserv.icors.org/SCRIPTS/WA-ICORS.
 EXE?A0=ADD_MED

Addiction Rehabilitation Facilities – www.arf.org/isd/bib/mental.html

Addiction Technology Transfer Center – www.nattc.org/index.html

Addiction Today – www.addictiontoday.org

ADDICT-L list – http://listserv.kent.edu/archives/addict-l.html

Alcohol and Alcohol Problems Science Database – http://etoh.niaaa.nih.gov/

Alcohol and Drug History Society – http://historyofalcoholanddrugs.typepad.com

Alcohol Concern (64 Leman Street, London, E1 8EU. Tel: 020 7264 0510; Fax: 020 7488
 9213; Email: contact@alcoholconcern.org.uk) – www.alcoholconcern.org.uk

Alcohol Drugs and Development – www.add-resources.org

Alcohol Focus Scotland – www.alcohol-focus-scotland.org.uk

Alcohol Misuse (Department of Health) – www.dh.gov.uk/en/Publichealth/
 Healthimprovement/Alcoholmisuse/index.htm

Alcohol Misuse list – www.jiscmail.ac.uk/lists/ALCOHOL-MISUSE.html

Alcohol, Other Drugs and Health: current evidence – www.bu.edu/aodhealth/index.html

Alcohol Policy Network – www.apolnet.ca/Index.html

Alcohol Reports – www.alcoholreports.blogspot.com

Alcoholics Anonymous – www.aa.org

Alcoholism and Substance Abuse Providers – www.asapnys.org

American Association of Colleges of Nursing. *Tool Kit for Cultural Competent
 Baccalaureate Nurses*; 2008. (This site will soon have a toolkit for graduate education as
 well.) – www.aacn.nche.edu/Education/pdf/toolkit.pdf

American Psychiatric Association – www.psych.org

American Society of Addiction Medicine – www.asam.org/CMEonline.html

ATTC Network – www.attcnetwork.org/index.asp

Australasian Professional Society on Alcohol and other Drugs – www.apsad.org.au/

Australian Drug Foundation – www.adf.org.au

Australian Drug Information Network – www.adin.com.au/content.asp?Document_ID=1

Australian Government Department of Health and Ageing

 Alcohol – www.alcohol.gov.au

 Illicit drugs – www.health.gov.au/internet/main/publishing.nsf/Content/health-
 pubhlth-strateg-drugs-illicit-index.htm

Mental health – www.health.gov.au/internet/main/publishing.nsf/Content/mental-pubs

Berman Institute of Bioethics – www.bioethicsinstitute.org

Best Practice Portal – www.emcdda.europa.eu/best-practice

BioMed Central – www.biomedcentral.com

Brain Injury Australia – www.bia.net.au

Brain Trauma Foundation – www.braintrauma.org

Brief Addiction Science Information Source (BASIS) – www.basisonline.org

Campaign for Effective Prevention and Treatment of Addiction – www.solutionstodrugs.com/index.htm

Centre for Addiction and Mental Health – www.camh.net

Centre for Clinical and Academic Workforce Innovation (Tel: 01623 819140; Email: ccawi@lincoln.ac.uk) – www.lincoln.ac.uk/ccawi

Centre for Evidence-based Mental Health (CEBMH) – www.cebmh.com

Centre for HIV and Sexual Health, Sheffield Primary Care NHS Trust – www.sexualhealthsheffield.nhs.uk

Centre for Independent Thought – www.centerforindependentthought.org

Centre for Mental Health – www.centreformentalhealth.org.uk

Clan Unity – www.clan-unity.co.uk

Committee on Publication Ethics – http://publicationethics.org

Communities of Practice for Local Government – www.communities.idea.gov.uk

Community Nursing Network– www.communitynursingnetwork.org

Co-morbid Mental Health and Substance Misuse in Scotland – www.scotland.gov.uk/Publications/2006/06/05104841/0)

Co-occurring Mental and Substance Abuse Disorders: a guide for mental health planning and advisory councils; 2003 – www.namhpac.org/PDFs/CO.pdf

Creative Commons – http://creativecommons.org

Cultural Competency in Health: a guide for policy, partnership and participation; 2005 – www.nhmrc.gov.au/_files_nhmrc/file/publications/synopses/hp19.pdf

Daily Dose: drug and alcohol news from around the world. (This website is no longer in continuous service, but the archives are still available.) – http://dailydose.net

Dartmouth Psychiatric Research Centre – www.dartmouth.edu/~prc

Database of Uncertainties about the Effects of Treatment – www.library.nhs.uk/DUETs/Default.aspx

Department of Health – www.dh.gov.uk

Department of Primary Health Care – www.primarycare.ox.ac.uk/research/dipex

Doctors.net.uk – www.doctors.org.uk

Double Trouble in Recovery: http://doubletroubleinrecovery.org

    A list of peer-reviewed journal articles on Double Trouble in Recovery: http://doubletroubleinrecovery.org/research.html

    Citations for biomedical literature published in peer-reviewed journals. Most citations resulting from a search for Double Trouble in Recovery link to the full text article: www.ncbi.nlm.nih.gov/pubmed

Drink and Drugs News – www.drinkanddrugs.net

Drinks Media Wire – www.drinksmediawire.com

Drug and Alcohol Findings – http://findings.org.uk

Drug and Alcohol Nurses of Australia – www.danaonline.org

Drug and Alcohol Services South Australia – www.dassa.sa.gov.au

Drug Day Programmes list – http://health.groups.yahoo.com/group/drug_day_programmes

DrugInfo Clearing House – http://druginfo.adf.org.au

Drug Misuse Information Scotland – www.drugmisuse.isdscotland.org

Drug Misuse Research list – www.jiscmail.ac.uk/lists/DRUG-MISUSE-RESEARCH.html

Drugs and Mental Health – www.thesite.org/drinkanddrugs/drugsafety/drugsandyourbody/drugsandmentalhealth

Drug Talk list – http://lists.sublimeip.com/mailman/listinfo/drugtalk

Drugtext Internet Library – www.drugtext.org

Dual Diagnosis – www.hoseahouse.org/infirmary/dualdx.html

Dual Diagnosis Australia and New Zealand – www.dualdiagnosis.org.au/home/

Dual Diagnosis Toolkit – www.rethink.org/dualdiagnosis/toolkit.html

Dual Diagnosis Website – http://users.erols.com/ksciacca

Enter Mental Health – www.entermentalhealth.net/home2.html

European Alcohol Policy Alliance – www.eurocare.org

European Association for the Treatment of Addiction – www.eata.org.uk

European Federation of Nurses Associations – www.efnweb.org/version1/en/index.html

European Monitoring Centre for Drugs and Drug Addiction – www.emcdda.europa.eu

European Working Group on Drugs Oriented Research – www.dass.stir.ac.uk/old-site/sections/scot-ad/ewodor.htm

Evidence-based Practice Web Sites – http://davisplus.fadavis.com/purnell/evidence_based_weblinks.cfm

Eye Movement Desensitisation and Reprocessing Training Workshops – www.emdrworkshops.com

Faces and Voices of Recovery – www.facesandvoicesofrecovery.org

Federation of Drug and Alcohol Professionals – www.fdap.org.uk/certification/dap.html

Gambling International list – http://health.groups.yahoo.com/group/GamblingIssuesInternational/

Global Alcohol Harm Reduction Network – http://groups.google.com/group/gahr-net

Global Health Council – www.globalhealth.org

Guardian UK. The most useful websites on dual diagnosis – http://society.guardian.co.uk/mentalhealth/page/0,8149,688817,00.html

Headway – www.headway.org.uk

Health and Safety Executive (HSE) – www.hse.gov.uk/stress

HIT – www.hit.org.uk

Horatio: European Psychiatric Nurses – www.horatio-web.eu

Hub of Commissioned Alcohol Projects and Policies (HubCAPP) (This is an online resource of local alcohol initiatives throughout England and Wales.) – www.hubcapp.org.uk

Inexcess: in search of recovery – www.inexcess.tv

International Brain Injury Association – www.internationalbrain.org

International Centre for Alcohol Policies – www.icap.org

International Council on Alcohol and Addictions – www.icaa.ch

International Council of Nurses – www.icn.ch

International Drug Policy Consortium – www.idpc.net

International Harm Reduction Association – www.ihra.net

International Network on Brief Interventions for Alcohol Problems (INEBRIA) – www.inebria.net

International Nurses Society on Addictions – www.intnsa.org

International Society of Addiction Journal Editors – www.parint.org/isajewebsite/index.htm

IVO: scientific institute in lifestyle, addiction and social developments – www.ivo.nl

James Lind Library – www.jameslindlibrary.org

Join Together: advancing effective alcohol and drug policy, prevention and treatment – www.jointogether.org

Links to Other Websites Related to Addiction – www.well.com/user/woa/aodsites.htm

Madness and Literature Network – www.madnessandliterature.org/index.php

Medical Council on Alcohol – www.m-c-a.org.uk

Medline Plus – www.nlm.nih.gov/medlineplus/dualdiagnosis.html

Mental Health (About.com) – http://mentalhealth.about.com

Mental Health and Addiction 101 (Centre for Addiction and Mental Health, Canada) – www.camh.net/MHA101/

Mental Health and Addictions Research Network – www.mhanet.ca/index.php

Mental Health Europe – www.mhe-sme.org/en.html

Mental Health Forum – www.mentalhealthforum.net/forum

Mental Health First Aid: Australia – www.mhfa.com.au

Mental Health First Aid: Canada – www.mentalhealthfirstaid.ca/Pages/default.aspx

Mental Health First Aid: England – www.mhfaengland.org.uk

Mental Health First Aid: Hong Kong – www.mhfa.org.hk

Mental Health First Aid: Scotland – www.smhfa.com

Mental Health First Aid: Singapore – www.mhfa.sg

Mental Health First Aid: South Africa – www.mhfasa.co.za/about.htm

Mental Health First Aid: USA – www.thenationalcouncil.org/cs/program_overview

Mental Health First Aid: Wales – www.mhfa-wales.org.uk

Mental Health Foundation – www.mentalhealth.org.uk/welcome

Mental Health Information for All (RCPSYCH) – www.rcpsych.ac.uk/mentalhealthinfoforall.aspx

Mental Health in Higher Education – www.mhhe.heacademy.ac.uk/sitepages/educators/?edid=239

Mental Health Policy Implementation Guide: dual diagnosis good practice guide (2002) – www.dh.gov.uk/en/Publicationsandstatistics/Publications/PublicationsPolicyAndGuidance/DH_4009058

Mental Health Research Network – http://homepages.ed.ac.uk/mhrn

Middlesex University Dual Diagnosis Courses – www.mdx.ac.uk/courses/postgraduate/nursing_midwifery_health/PGCert_Dual_Diagnosis.aspx

MIND – www.mind.org.uk

Ministry of Justice (National Offender Management Service) – www.justice.gov.uk/about/noms.htm

Mood Disorders Association of Canada – www.mooddisorderscanada.ca

Motivational Interventions for Drugs and Alcohol Misuse in Schizophrenia – www.midastrial.ac.uk

Motivational Interviewing – www.motivationalinterview.org

National Alliance on Mental Illness – www.nami.org

National Centre for Education and Training on Addiction – www.nceta.flinders.edu.au/index.html

National Comorbidity Initiative – www.health.gov.au/internet/main/publishing.nsf/Content/health-pubhlth-publicat-document-metadata-comorbidity.htm

National Consortium of Consultant Nurses in Dual Diagnosis and Substance Use – www.dualdiagnosis.co.uk

National Drug and Alcohol Research Centre – http://ndarc.med.unsw.edu.au/

National Drug Research Institute – http://ndri.curtin.edu.au

National Health Service – www.nhs.uk

National Health Service Litigation Authority – www.nhsla.com/home.htm

National Institute on Alcohol Abuse and Alcoholism (NIAAA) (5635 Fishers Lane, MSC 9304, Bethesda, MD 20892-9304, USA; Tel: 301-443-3860; Email: www.niaaa.nih.gov/ContactUs.htm) – www.niaaa.nih.gov

National Institute on Drug Abuse, National Institutes of Health (6001 Executive Boulevard, Room 5213, Bethesda, MD 20892-9561, USA; Tel: 301-443-1124, Email: information@nida.nih.gov) – www.nida.nih.gov

National Institute for Health and Clinical Excellence (MidCity Place, 71 High Holborn, London, WC1V 6NA, UK; Tel: 0845 003 7780; Fax: 0845 003 7784; Email: nice@nice.org.uk) – www.nice.org.uk

National Institute of Mental Health – www.nimh.nih.gov

National Quality Forum (This site primarily focuses on organizational cultural competence.) – www.qualityforum.org/Search.aspx?keyword=cultural+c0mpetent+organizations

National Registry of Evidence-Based Programs (NREPP): Double Trouble in Recovery (2007) www.nrepp.samhsa.gov/ViewIntervention.aspx?id=13

National Treatment Agency for Substance Misuse – www.nta.nhs.uk

New Directions in the Study of Alcohol – www.newdirections.org.uk

New South Wales Health Dual Disorders resources – www.druginfo.nsw.gov.au/illicit_drugs

NHS CHOICES – www.nhs.uk/conditions/heat-exhaustion-and-heatstroke/Pages/Introduction.aspx

NHS Institute for Innovation and Improvement – www.institute.nhs.uk

Nordic Council on Dual Diagnosis – www.norden.org/en/areas-of-co-operation/alcohol-and-drugs

O'Grady CP, Skinner WJ. *Family Guide to Concurrent Disorders* (2007) – www.camh.net/publications/resources_for_professionals/partnering_with_families/partnering_families_famguide.pdf

Partnership in Coping – www.pinc-recovery.com

PROGRESS: National Consortium of Consultant Nurses in Dual Diagnosis and Substance Use – www.dualdiagnosis.co.uk

Promoting Adult Learning – www.niace.org.uk/current-work/area/mental-health

Psychiatric Nursing – www.citypsych.com/index.html

Psychminded – www.psychminded.co.uk

Public Access (National Institutes of Health) – http://publicaccess.nih.gov/index.htm

Rethink (UK) – www.rethink.org/dualdiagnosis

Royal College of General Practitioners – www.rcgp.org.uk

Royal College of Psychiatrists – www.rcpsych.ac.uk

Royal Society for the Encouragement of Arts – www.thersa.org/home

Sainsbury Centre for Mental Health – www.scmh.org.uk/index.aspx

SANE Australia – www.sane.org

Schizophrenia Society of Canada – www.schizophrenia.ca

Scholarship Society – www.scholarshipsociety.org

Scottish Addiction Studies – www.dass.stir.ac.uk/sections/showsection.php?id=4

Scottish Addiction Studies Library – www.drugslibrary.stir.ac.uk

Social Care Institute for Excellence – www.scie.org.uk

Social Care Online – www.scie-socialcareonline.org.uk

Society for the Study of Addiction – www.addiction-ssa.org

Spanish Peaks Mental Health Centre – www.spmhc.org

Stigma in Mental Health and Addiction – www.cmhanl.ca/pdf/Stigma.pdf

Substance Abuse and Mental Health Center – Toolkit for integrated treatment for co-occurring disorders – http://store.samhsa.gov/shin/content/SMA08-4367/SMA08-4367-01.pdf and www.nebhands.nebraska.edu/files/Integrated%20Treatment%20information%20for%20Consumers.pdf

Substance Abuse and Mental Health Data Archive – www.icpsr.umich.edu/SAMHDA/

Substance Abuse and Mental Health Services Administration – www.samhsa.gov

Substance Misuse Management in General Practice – www.smmgp.org.uk

The Addiction Project – www.theaddictionproject.com

The Clifford Beers Foundation: *The Promotion of Mental Health*, vol. 1 (1992) – www.cliffordbeersfoundation.co.uk/jcont91.htm

The Co-occurring Centre of Excellence (US) – www.coce.samhsa.gov

The European Monitoring Centre for Drugs and Drug Addiction: www.emcdda.europa.eu

The International Community for Hearing Voices – www.intervoiceonline.org

The International Network of Nurses – www.tinnurses.org

The International Society for the Study of Drug Policy – www.issdp.org

The James Lind Alliance Guidebook – www.jlaguidebook.org

The Management Standards Consultancy – www.themsc.org

The Mentor Foundation – www.mentorfoundation.org/

The Methadone Alliance – www.m-alliance.org.uk/forum.html

The National Centre on Addiction and Substance Abuse – www.casacolumbia.org/templates/Home.aspx?articleid=287&zoneid=32

The National Comorbidity Initiative (Australia) – www.health.gov.au/internet/publishing.nsf/Content?national-comorbidity-initiative-2

The National Drug and Alcohol Research Centre – http://ndarc.med.unsw.edu.au

The National Institute on Drug Abuse – www.drugabuse.gov/nidahome.html

The National Treatment Agency – www.nta.nhs.uk

The Recovery Workshop – www.recoveryworkshop.com

The Royal College of Psychiatrists: Changing Minds campaign – www.rcpsych.ac.uk/campaigns/previouscampaigns/changingminds.aspx

The Sacred Space Foundation – www.sacredspace.org.uk

The Tidal Model – www.tidal-model.com

The Wellcome Centre for Neuroethics – www.neuroethics.ox.ac.uk

Therapeutic Communities list – www.jiscmail.ac.uk/lists/THERAPEUTIC-COMMUNITIES.html

Think Cultural Health: bridging the health care gap through cultural competence continuing education. (This site, developed by the US Department of Minority Health has continuing education modules for physicians, nurses and other healthcare providers, and the Health Care Languages Implementation Guide.) – www.thinkculturalhealth.org and https://hclsig.thinkculturalhealth.hhs.gov

Tilburg University, Department of Tranzo – www.uvt.nl/tranzo

Toc H – www.tochparticipation.co.uk

Treatment Improvement Exchange – www.treatment.org

Trimbos Institute: Netherlands institute of mental health and addiction – www.trimbos.org

Turning Point – www.turning-point.co.uk

Tx Director – www.txdirector.com

UK Drug Policy Commission – www.ukdpc.org.uk/index.shtml

United Nations Office on Drugs and Crime – www.unodc.org

University of Toronto Joint Centre for Bioethics Centre for Addiction and Mental Health Bioethics Service – www.jointcentreforbioethics.ca/partners/camh.shtml

UNGASS (United Nations General Assembly Special Session on the World Drug Problem) – www.ungassondrugs.org

Update: an alcohol and other drugs information bulletin board – http://lists.sublimeip.com/mailman/listinfo/update

Victorian Alcohol and Drug Association – www.vaada.org.au

Wired In to Recovery: empowering people to tackle substance use problems – http://wiredin.org.uk

World Health Organization: Climate change and human health – www.who.int/globalchange/en

World Health Organization: Management of substance abuse – www.who.int/substanceabuse/en

World Health Organization: Mental health – www.who.int/mental_health/policy/en

World Medical Association – www.wma.net/en/10home/index.html

Youth Drug Support, Australia – www.yds.org.au

Youth Health Talk – www.youthtalkonline.com

Index